L.B of Redbridge

THE GOOD HAIR GUIDE:
ALL YOUR QUESTIONS
ANSWERED

THE GOOD HAIR GUIDE: ALL YOUR QUESTIONS ANSWERED

Vanessa Bailey

Book Guild Publishing
Sussex, England

First published in Great Britain in 2007 by
The Book Guild Ltd
Pavilion View
19 New Road
Brighton, BN1 1UF

Copyright © Vanessa Bailey 2007

The right of Vanessa Bailey to be identified as the author of this work has been asserted by her in accordance with the Copyright, Designs and Patents Act 1988.

All rights reserved. No part of this publication may be reproduced, transmitted, or stored in a retrieval system, in any form, or by any means, without permission in writing from the publisher, nor be otherwise circulated in any form of binding or cover other than that in which it is published and without a similar condition being imposed on the subsequent purchaser.

Typesetting in Times by
SetSystems Ltd, Saffron Walden, Essex

Printed in Great Britain by
CPI Bath

A catalogue record for this book is
available from the British Library

ISBN 978 84624 119 2

Contents

	Foreword	vii
	Acknowledgements	ix
	Introduction	1
1	Male Hair Loss	3
2	Female Hair Loss	15
3	Children's Hair	37
4	Afro-Caribbean Hair	47
5	General Hair and Scalp Facts	57
6	Myths	79
7	Useful Contacts	87
	Index	89

Foreword

In our Western culture, those with hair or scalp problems may consult a variety of specialists such as a retail pharmacist, a hairdresser, a trichologist, a general medical practitioner or a dermatologist – and many others! During the last 25 years, several comprehensive textbooks have been written, providing detailed information for such specialists and their clients in the 'World of Hair'.

This succinct, well-illustrated and detailed book combines some aspects of most areas of hair and scalp aesthetics and science; a very good source of information for both the general public and the trichologist. It is 'different' and particularly useful because of the way it is presented – basically written as Vanessa Bailey's professional answers to almost 100 of the commonest questions that clients ask during their consultation.

Dr. R.P.R. Dawber MA.FRCP

Acknowledgements

I wish to thank Dr Rodney Dawber for reading my script and for allowing me the use of his fantastic photographs of hair and scalp disorders. Having studied from Dr Dawber's books on hair and scalp problems as a student trichologist and having read all his books published since on the subject, it was indeed an honour to receive from him such positive feedback, encouragement and advice with this project.

My thanks to Dr Bessam Farjo for the use of his hair transplant photographs, clearly showing an example of such high professional standards being achieved in this area of expertise.

My thanks also go to the proofreaders at The Institute of Trichologists. And finally, I would also like to thank my brother Graham and sister Felicity for reading my script and for all their valued comments.

trichology *n.* **the study of the hair and scalp and their diseases** – **trichologist** *n.*

Oxford English Dictionary 2004

Introduction

When I decided to put this project together, my initial thoughts were solely of directing it at the hair-suffering general public. I thought a question and answer book would be an easy to use reference format, information would hopefully be easily found somewhere throughout for just about anyone with a hair loss problem and the reader would be able to quickly relate to a myriad of hair worries that only they thought they had. At the very least I thought it may prompt someone who perhaps hadn't heard of trichology before to make contact with The Institute of Trichologists and get put in touch with a professional.

Although I still wish for this book to remain firmly within the general public domain, as this project developed I began to realise, or at least hoped, that student trichologists and newly-qualified trichologists may also benefit from this book in a practical way. Text displayed in this fashion using real client questions, 'real language' and real-life case histories should help marry-up newly acquired knowledge with everyday practice. All experienced trichologists must remember what a lonely transition it can be, moving from textbook to consulting room.

Whether you plan to seek help for a hair

problem, are about to qualify or have just qualified as a trichologist, I really hope you find trichological knowledge displayed in this format refreshing and helpful.

1
Male Hair Loss

Men who happen to be genetically predisposed towards hair loss often notice the first signs of thinning between the ages of eighteen and twenty-five; hairline recession and widening of the crown area are quickly apparent. However, men with disposable incomes and perhaps a little extra time on their hands are now able to take advantage of the results of recent scientific research (take a look at Question 5; approved lotions and tablets are noted here). Surgical hair transplant methods are advancing all the time too; long gone are the 'dolls head' punch graft techniques of twenty or thirty years ago. Sophisticated 'micro grafting' is common practice and creates natural looking results (Question 11 explains hair transplantation and illustrates the results commonly achieved today).

Male Pattern Baldness (androgenetic alopecia): A Little Piece of Science

In the genetically predisposed, hair follicles (tube or sock-like openings of skin where hair develops) positioned along the front hairline, across the top of the scalp and all the way back to the crown are sensitive to male hormones, in particular, dihydrotestosterone (DHT).

Testosterone is converted to potent DHT by an enzyme called 5 alpha reductase (whose activity has been found to be higher in balding than in non-balding men).

Once exposed to DHT, hair growth reduces as these follicles miniaturise and thinner and shorter hairs are produced until only tiny, colourless hairs remain. These miniature hairs are known as vellus hairs. Even on an apparently bald scalp, upon close examination a layer of vellus hair often remains visible, that is unless the follicles give up completely and allow the shiny bald situation to arise.

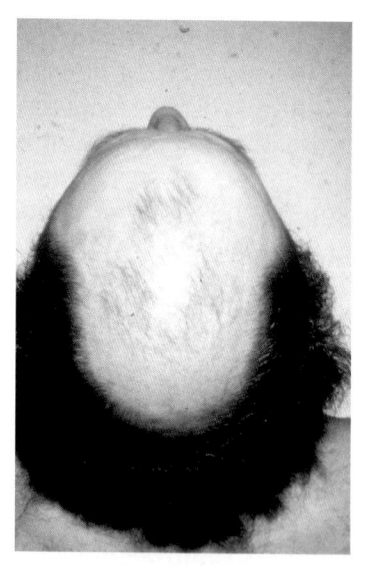

Male Pattern Baldness
Photograph courtesy of Dr R. Dawber

Q1 I suffer with hereditary male hair loss, am I right to assume that I have inherited this from my father's side of the family?

Not necessarily, hereditary hair thinning can be passed on from either side of the family.

Q2 I am a fifty-five-year-old male with a full head of hair: do you think I could still go completely bald?

You are one of the lucky ones! If you were genetically programmed to suffer complete loss of hair from the top of your scalp it would have been evident by now (see Question 4), although you may notice a little hair thinning as you get older.

Q3 I am completely bald on top. While I'm on holiday how can I prevent the top of my head from getting sunburnt without having to wear a cap all the time?

Sun creams or blocks that you would normally use on your face and body can be applied to your scalp; choose the spray-on varieties for easy application and choose at least a factor 25 for the highly exposed scalp area. These products decrease the chances of developing sunburn and potential skin malignancies.

Individuals with only slight hair loss and those with tinted, bleached or highlighted hair should also be careful in sunny climates; see Question 26 (part H).

Q4 How old are the majority of men when they finally experience complete baldness?

On average, if a complete loss of hair from the top of the scalp is determined, it usually strikes between thirty and sixty years of age.

Q5 Are there any treatments on the market for male pattern hair loss?

To date, there are two licensed hair loss treatments available: Regaine (minoxidil) by Pfizer, also known as Rogaine in the USA, and Propecia (finasteride), UK and USA by Merck.

Minoxidil was originally taken in tablet form to reduce high blood pressure and was found (by side-effect) to promote increased hair growth. Subsequently, it was licensed as a topical (scalp applied) hair loss treatment.

Minoxidil may hold hairs that are just about to pass into the telogen (resting) phase (from where they will be shed), in the anagen (active growth) phase (see Question 15 where the hair growth cycle is explained). Minoxidil may also strengthen existing hair growth and may encourage some new hair growth too.

Propecia (finasteride) is an orally administered medically prescribed drug and is the latest known treatment for male hair loss. Just as with minoxidil, finasteride was found to be a hair treatment by mistake. It was originally used to treat disorders of the prostate gland (and still is). These patients noticed that their previously thinning crown areas started to appear thicker while taking this drug. Therefore, a reduced dose is now in use for male pattern baldness sufferers.

Finasteride inhibits the action of the 5-alpha reductase enzyme; this leads to a reduction in DHT while hardly affecting testosterone levels. There is a very slight chance that this treatment may cause some loss of libido but this clears once the drug is discontinued. Finasteride may slow the progression of male pattern hair loss, strengthen existing hair growth and could promote some new hair growth too.

In essence, both of these treatments need to be administered before complete baldness occurs to stand a chance of gaining an appreciable cosmetic difference. For individuals suffering the effects of the later stages of male pattern baldness a more drastic approach may be investigated. Depending on the individual case in hand, surgical hair replacement may be of benefit (see Question 11); alternatively non-surgical hair replacement may be preferred.

Non-surgical hair replacement involves wearing a fine mesh or net. This mesh is secured onto the scalp by special adhesives. Attached to the mesh is either human or synthetic hair, depending on what is preferred and what is easiest for the individual concerned to style and maintain. Therefore, this is in essence a form of hairpiece; beware of sharp salesmen claiming that it is not and that the hair will grow from the scalp itself!

Refer also to Question 64, which deals with cover-up sprays and hair mascaras. These products disguise areas of the scalp exposed by hair thinning.

Remember, before embarking on any treatment, obtain the advice of a qualified trichologist (see Chapter 7). Correct diagnosis is paramount at the outset to determine the cause of your hair loss problem. (There are other forms of hair loss apart from hereditary baldness, as you will see further on into this book. Other forms of hair loss require other forms of treatment, or simply just plain sound advice.) A qualified trichologist will ultimately save you time, money and false hope.

Q6 Once you start a treatment regime for male pattern hair loss, can you ever come off it?

If you decided to stop treatment, this is fine, but you will notice that any cosmetic improvements gained will begin to fade. Even the tried and tested treatments, (Regaine and Propecia), are not true 'cures'. Therefore, continuous use is necessary to achieve and maintain any positive results.

Q7 My friend has heard that it is possible to apply Regaine and take Propecia at the same time; is this true?

Yes, this is possible. See Question 5: Regaine seems to prolong the anagen or active growth phase of the hair growth cycle and Propecia reduces DHT levels. With combined use you may therefore achieve better results.

Q8 I have heard that castration is the only cure for male pattern baldness, is this true?

Ideally this would need to be carried out before puberty for maximum effect; halting testosterone production in the first place would prevent the testosterone-dihydrotestosterone-follicle attack process from occurring (see pages 3–4 for further technical details). However, if male pattern baldness is already apparent in an adult male and castration was performed, dead hair follicles would not be brought back to life. Nothing can bring back hair that has already been lost.

Q9 Is it true that scientists have discovered the baldness gene?

The gene responsible for a hair loss condition termed as alopecia universalis (complete loss of scalp and body hair) has been discovered. However, the gene(s) responsible for androgenetic alopecia (common pattern baldness) remains elusive.

Q10 I am an eighteen-year-old-male. I do not have any specific problems with my hair but I would like to get into some healthy hair care habits now while I am still young, any ideas?

You are very wise, although this is a common request nowadays. It seems men are becoming as particular about grooming as women, especially amongst the younger generations. It is true that the application of simple yet effective tips on caring for your hair can make an immense difference to its health and therefore outward appearance. Reference can be made to the following points raised in this book (hair loss sufferers should take note too):

- Shampoo technique and frequency: see Questions 65 and 72.
- The application of hair conditioners: see Question 65.
- Diet advice. Feed those follicles! Take a look at Question 75.
- When is it best to comb or brush your hair (separate rules apply to wet and dry hair) and what types of combs and brushes are healthiest? Take a look at Questions 73 and 74.

Q11 What is actually involved during hair transplantation procedures?

Micro grafting is the latest state-of-the-art hair transplant technique widely used by today's skilled hair surgeons.

Under local anaesthetic, a strip of hairy skin is surgically removed form the back or sides of the scalp (this is the 'donor site'). Compared to the hair follicles on the top of the scalp, the follicles of the donor site are not genetically programmed to wither, and are independent of the area of scalp they are transferred to. This piece of skin is then delicately separated into micrografts that contain between just one and three hairs (useful for creating natural-looking hair lines), and mini grafts that contain between four and eight hairs (useful for adding bulk to larger areas of baldness, such as the crown). Micro grafting therefore replaces the old-style plug or punch grafting technique, whereby grafts contained far too many hairs and the 'doll's head' look was invariably created (see the pictures on the following page illustrating the results of today's techniques).

Three months following surgery the first signs of hair growth appear, however, in most cases an individual will need more than one session to achieve an ideal level of density, depending of course on the quantity and the quality of hair that grows from the donor site. Remember the hair that was removed from the donor site will not grow back again. In essence you are relocating the hair that you have, rather than actually gaining additional hair growth; it's a case of redistribution rather than regeneration. When appropriate, qualified trichologists offer referrals to reputable hair transplant surgeons.

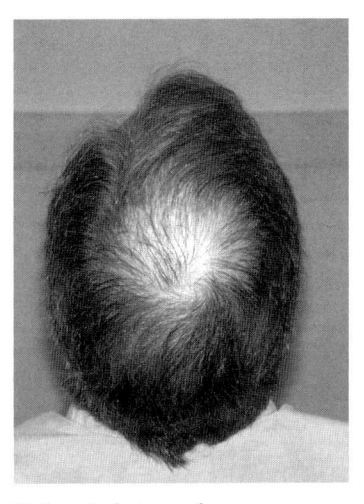

Before hair transplant surgery
Photographs courtesy of Dr B. Farjo

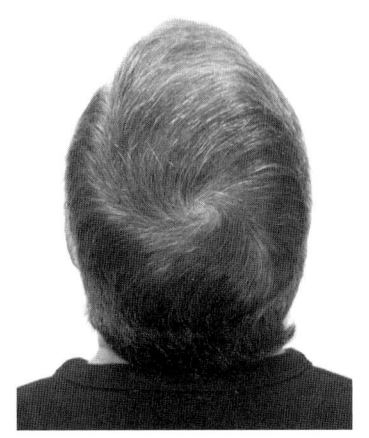

After hair transplant surgery

Q12 I am considering a hair transplant, can you still cut, style and even dye the transplanted hair?

Yes, you can carry on as normal with transplanted hair. This hair is exactly the same in structure and form as when it was growing from its original site. Just ensure that you use a hair-conditioning product after every shampoo (take a look at Question 26).

Q13 I am a thirty-eight-year-old male and have a receding hairline. However, just recently I have noticed a definite increase in the amount of hair stuck to my comb and all over my pillow in the mornings. Does this mean my inherited hair thinning condition is progressing?

To help rule out advancing pattern loss, ask yourself the following questions: have you suffered a severe bout of stress during the last six months? Have you suffered an illness in the last six months that resulted in a high fever? (See the list of common causes of hair loss on page 20). Have you been prescribed any medication lately? (See page 21; particular drugs are highlighted here that are known to temporarily disturb the hair growth cycle.) Have you been through a period of erratic eating patterns recently? If this is the case see Question 75 for a list of 'hair foods' to include in your diet regularly and avoid skipping meals.

If you answered yes to any of the above questions, the good news here is that this type of hair shedding should ease up and the hair lost through such changes in your system should start to re-grow over the following six-month period (see page 19, in particular the section entitled 'Acute telogen effluvium'). It is also recommended that you ask your doctor to carry out a simple blood test to check your thyroid function and iron levels (see page 21, parts F and G).

Q14 I have been recommended administration of DHEA (dehydroepiandrosterone) by a friend of mine to improve my overall well-being and mental alertness. Seeing as DHEA has been thought of as an anti-ageing treatment, could it help my thinning hair?

DHEA is one of a group of steroid hormones naturally produced by the adrenal glands. The adrenal glands are endocrine glands (glands that secrete hormones directly into the bloodstream). They are found above each kidney and from here they produce hormones that regulate glucose metabolism, salt balance, male hormones and those 'fight or flight' hormones that enable the body to react appropriately during stress.

However, back to DHEA, which is considered a weak androgen or male-like hormone. However, once secreted into the blood it can be converted into the powerful male hormone testosterone.

DHEA declines naturally with age and claims have surfaced that DHEA is an anti-ageing hormone. However, supplementing DHEA levels in ageing men (and women) does not necessarily mean a return to the wonders of youth. During double blind trails,[1,2] administration of DHEA-S (a form of DHEA) improved the sense of well-being, libido (particularly in women) and skin health in terms of hydration and thickness in some (but not in all) of the individuals tested. Another study also found a slight increase in testosterone levels in individuals prescribed DHEA.[3]

In relation to your thinning hair an increase in testosterone levels through taking DHEA could make matters worse. I would feel therefore that it is wise to seek medical advice before taking any such medication and, if prescribed DHEA, never exceed your recommended dose.

PLEASE NOTE: Currently DHEA is not licensed for use in the UK.

Notes

1 **Yen SSC, Morales AJ, Khorram O *et al.*** (1995) Replacement of DHEA in aging men and women, *Ann. NY Acad Sci.* 774: 128–42.
2 **Flynn MA, Weaver-Osterholtz D, Sharpe-Timms KL**

et al. (1999) Dehydroepiandrosterone replacement in aging humans, *J. Clin. Endocrinol. Metab*, 84: 1527–33.
3 **Baulieu EE, Thomas G, Legrain S *et al.*** (2000) Dehydroepiandrosterone (DHEA), DHEA sulfate, and ageing: contribution of the DHEAge study to a sociobiomedical issue, *Proc. Natl. Acad. Sci. USA*, 97: 4279–84.

2

Female Hair Loss

There is a widespread notion that only men lose their hair, but most women, if not all women by old age, do at some point experience hair changes of some degree during their lives. Another issue is social acceptance; the world is far more accepting of men suffering hair loss. It is far easier for a man with thinning hair to simply decide to shave it all off and forget about it and still look good (and even fashionable), but no such psychology or fashion exists for women.

It is therefore vitally important to set out the causes of female hair loss. Many issues will be discussed throughout this chapter, and a lot of helpful advice will be given via questions from a broad spectrum of women, covering a wide age span.

However, before the 'question and answer' section begins, a little background information is required. Firstly, female pattern baldness or female androgenetic alopecia will be explored. This is the most common hair loss complaint found among women.

Female Pattern Baldness (female androgenetic alopecia)

Just like male pattern baldness, the female version is also a genetic condition; hair follicles are deemed locally sensitive, once again, to 'male' hormones without there necessarily being an increase in hormone levels. However, the 'patterns' of thinning are distinct. With women, the thinning usually appears just behind the front hairline (leaving the front hairline intact), then gradually spreads across the top of the scalp back towards the crown. Fortunately, complete baldness is a rarity among women.

Refer to the photograph showing a case of male pattern baldness on page 4 and to the photograph on the following page of female androgenetic alopecia/ female pattern baldness and compare the slight differences in form. However, it has to be said that some post-menopausal women develop hair loss in the distinctive male pattern.

Female androgenetic alopecia is considered slower in progression than the male version. However, as in male hair loss, due to a gradual reduction in the size of the hair follicles (in the affected region of scalp), the subsequent reduction in length and, in particular, diameter of each hair will encourage greater exposure of the scalp or widening of the partings.

Female androgenetic alopecia most often affects women around the time of the menopause (see Question 18), but it can be genetically determined to appear any time following puberty. It is also known that if a particular medical problem were to occur or if certain prescribed drugs were administered that managed to exert an androgenic (male-type) effect on the system, then an existing case of female androgenetic alopecia

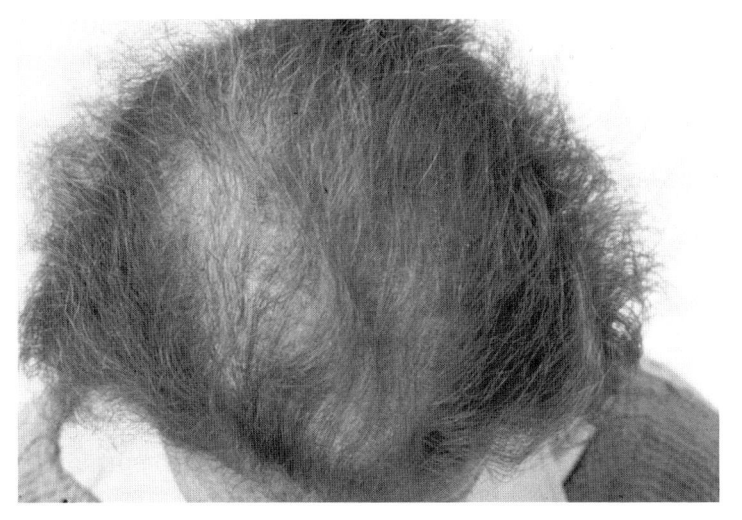

Female pattern baldness/female androgenetic alopecia
Photograph courtesy of Dr R. Dawber

may be negatively affected or possibly induced in the genetically predisposed. Here are the most common of these interfering scenarios, found in particular among premenopausal women:

Polycystic ovarian syndrome (PCOS)

This medical condition results in the body producing increased quantities of androgens (so-called male hormones). Hirsutism (this describes an increase in hair growth on the face and the body), acne, menstrual problems and weight gain are all symptoms of PCOS.

Among other treatments, women who suffer PCOS are commonly medically prescribed anti-androgens (drugs that aim to inhibit the action of androgens or male-like hormones). Under such circumstances women who suffer androgenetic alopecia may find anti-androgens helpful with regard to scalp hair health (see Question 22 for current treatment regimes available for female androgenetic alopecia).

PLEASE NOTE: PCOS requires medical attention.

Progestogen-only and high strength combined oral contraceptives

Natural progesterone (a hormone produced by the ovaries) and its synthetic counterparts are collectively known as progestogens. However, some of the synthetic counterparts are hair negative. In particular, progestogen-only and high strength combined oral contraceptives predominately contain either norethisterone or norgestrel, which have androgenic or male-like activity. Norethisterone and norgestrel are also used in some progestogen-only contraceptive injections and implants as well as some hormone replacement preparations (menopausal women should refer to Question 16).

The standard strength combined oral contraceptive pill Dianette (see also Question 22) contains a decidedly hair-positive anti-androgen. Or some of the other standard or lower strength combined pills such as Yasmin and Marvelon that contain either desogestrel or gestodene as the progestogen are preferred alternatives for women already suffering androgenetic alopecia or for women who feel they may be susceptible to this condition. *Always seek medical advice on all types of hormone-acting contraceptives before use.*

We've investigated 'genetically programmed' hair loss. However, there are a host of other reasons why hair loss may occur, particularly in women. These conditions can be described as indicative of 'non-pattern hair loss'.

Non-pattern Hair Loss

Due to a variety of causes (see pages 20 and 21) the hair growth cycle (see Question 15) can be interrupted at any time of life. Such interruptions result in a sudden bout of excessive hair shedding that allows for an overall reduction in hair density, although in the case of anagen effluvium (see below) a complete loss of hair can occur. Non-pattern hair loss or hair loss not conforming to the distinct pattern of androgenetic alopecia is usually reversible and is further specified according to which stage of the hair growth cycle the interruption occurred.

Anagen effluvium

This describes hair being lost in the anagen (or active growth) phase. Hair is dramatically shed within days of exposure to a specific causative factor, such as, for example, the administration of chemotherapy (see Question 60). Although this condition can cause extensive or even complete loss of hair very quickly, the outcome is still a positive one. When exposure to the causative factor is removed, hair re-growth is rapid.

Acute telogen effluvium

This describes an increased mass of hair prematurely reaching the telogen or resting phase. On average up to a hundred telogen hairs are shed on a daily basis (see page 22 under the heading 'Telogen phase');

during telogen effluvium this number can increase considerably.

This type of heavy, visible shedding of hair typically occurs three to four months after the occurrence of a specific causative event such as, for example, a very high temperature, an extreme shock or a massive sudden weight loss. This cycle of dramatic hair shedding will persist for about three months, then hair re-growth will follow.

Chronic telogen effluvium

Sometimes telogen effluvium does not rectify itself as quickly as it should; chronic telogen effluvium is recognised when heavy hair shedding persists longer than six months as opposed to the usual three-month period. There is no known cause. This condition is often found in middle-aged women.

Common causes of non-pattern hair loss

A **Poor diet.** For example, regularly *skipping meals* or *general poor nutrition uptake.*
B **Shock and stress.** For example, *bereavement* or *serious injury* such as that sustained in a *serious car crash.* Although **acute telogen effluvium** most commonly occurs following these incidences, predisposed individuals may suffer a patchy hair loss condition termed as **alopecia areata.** (See Question 69).
C **Childbirth.** See Question 15.
D **Illness.** Including very high temperatures above 103°F.
E **Surgery.** Apart from the 'physical stress' of an operation, general anesthetics may temporarily interrupt the hair growth cycle.

F **Iron-deficiency (with or without anaemia).** Hair loss will be continuous unless this is corrected (see Question 20).

G **Hypothyroidism and severe hyperthyroidism.** The thyroid gland is one of our major endocrine glands (a gland that directly secretes hormones into the bloodstream). It produces the hormone thyroxine and actively controls our metabolism (the process by which the body utilises the food we eat). However, if the thyroid gland becomes under-(hypo) active or severely over-(hyper) active then hair loss may occur and be continuous unless the thyroid problems are corrected.

Some prescribed drugs may also cause hair loss (which is reversible on withdrawal). Common examples of these are:

- anti-blood clotting drugs;
- anti-depressants (long-term use);
- oral administration of a retinoid (a regime employed to treat severe cases of acne);
- antibiotics (long-term use);
- anti-cancer drugs (see page 19 under the section entitled 'Anagen Effluvium' and Question 60).

Q15 I had a baby three months ago and I am sure that my hair is coming out a little more than before. Could I be imagining this? If not, could I go completely bald?

You are not imagining it, but the good news is that you will not go completely bald, far from it. Due to elevated oestrogen (female hormone) levels during pregnancy, the usual daily shedding of around one hundred telogen hairs practically grinds to a halt (see below, where the hair growth cycle is explained). However, these 'collected or stored' hairs need to be released at some point in time and this is most commonly noticed three months after giving birth. The shedding will continue for a period of several months, after which hair regrowth will follow as your normal hair growth cycle re-establishes itself.

The Hair Growth Cycle

Hair follicles are continually passing through phases of active growth and rest. These phases are as follows:

Anagen phase

This is the active growth phase of the hair follicle where a hair can grow uninterrupted for up to six years. Normally 85 per cent or more of scalp hairs are in this phase at any given time.

Catagen phase

This is the transition phase of the hair growth cycle that follows the anagen but precedes the telogen phase. This phase lasts for around seven days and 1 per cent of scalp hairs should be in this phase at any given time.

Telogen phase

This is the resting phase of the hair growth cycle. At the end of this phase the hair is shed which constitutes the natural fall of up to a hundred hairs on a daily basis. The telogen phase normally lasts for around three months and under normal circumstances 14 per cent of scalp hairs should be in this phase at any given time. The shed hair will be replaced automatically as the hair follicles enter the anagen phase all over again. The hair growth cycle will continue to repeat itself thereafter.

Q16 I have been recommended by my GP to start taking hormone replacement therapy for the menopause. Will this thicken my thinning hair?

The menopause is a time when most women notice a change in their hair quality, be it just a little dryer than normal, lifeless, or in the worst case scenario actually thinning out. Woman who possess a genetic predisposition towards hair thinning are more likely to notice the latter. These problems surface due to the drop in oestrogen production.

The most common form of 'attack' on the symptoms of the menopause is the use of hormone replacement therapy (HRT). It is doubtful that HRT directly thickens hair or reverses hair loss, but any boost in flagging oestrogen levels is not a bad thing. Hair can feel softer, look shinier and be bouncier on HRT and some women even report stability in their hair thinning problems as well. If you require a progestogen (a collective term used to describe natural and synthetic forms of the hormone progesterone), as well as an oestrogen, avoid a regime that uses either norethisterone or norgestrel as the progestogen. These have androgenic (or male-like) activity and may therefore be detrimental to your thinning hair. See pages 16–18; note in particular the section entitled 'Progestogen-only and high strength combined oral contraceptives'. It would be advised that you ask your doctor about the possibility of using either medroxyprogesterone acetate or natural progesterone (e.g. Cyclogest) instead.

However, an HRT preparation that currently isn't available in the UK but would be worth enquiring about through your GP is Climen. This is the only HRT formulation to contain cyproterone acetate, which as discussed in Question 22, is an anti-androgen and could therefore be decidedly hair-positive.

PLEASE NOTE: Always seek medical advice on all types of HRT before use.

Q17 Both my sister and I are going through the menopause. I have noticed that my hair has thinned considerably, especially on the top of my scalp, but my sister's hair is practically as thick as before. If hormone changes can cause hair loss, why hasn't my sister's hair behaved like mine?

This is all down to genetics. If you happen to be genetically predisposed towards hair thinning, the drop in oestrogen production and the subsequent domination of male hormones at your time of life may result in this problem. Although you and your sister are experiencing similar hormone changes, if she is free from the genetic coding that decides hair thinning, it is unlikely that her hair will change as much.

Q18 How old are the majority of women when they begin to suffer the effects of female pattern baldness?

Most women first notice the start of this type of hair thinning when they are around forty-five to fifty years of age.

Q19 Considering all age groups, what percentage of women are affected by female pattern hair loss?

Before forty-five years of age up to 25 per cent of the female population suffer genetic hair thinning. This percentage climbs to 50 per cent between the ages of forty-five and seventy, but most of these cases are not obvious to the onlooker, just to the women themselves.

Q20 I am twenty-three and have been diagnosed as suffering iron-deficiency anaemia. Could this explain why my hair has been shedding a lot lately and is feeling thinner than it used to be? If so, will it grow back when I am better?

Iron-deficiency anaemia is a common cause of non-pattern hair loss amongst young women. See pages 19–21 where non-pattern hair loss is explained. Apart from other possible causes, iron-deficiency anaemia may result from the effects of menstruation and/or a diet lacking in iron-rich foods, (see Question 75 where examples of iron-containing foods are listed). Poor diet practices such as those highlighted on page 20 (part A) will increase susceptibility towards developing iron-deficiency anaemia. However, under most circumstances, once this condition has been corrected and if this is the sole reason for your hair loss problem, then hair re-growth will occur.

Under medical guidance, courses of iron supplements are usually recommended to correct a deficiency. Note that the stabilisation of hair shedding and the start of hair re-growth will not occur until three months after your iron levels have reached their peak. Therefore, in most cases, it may take at least six months before an initial reduction in hair shedding is noticed and a little longer again before hair re-growth is apparent. (Resist the temptation of not completing a full course of iron supplements due to frustration at not noticing an immediate reduction in hair loss.)

You should have an annual blood test to check for any signs of a relapse and maintain as healthy a diet as possible for both a healthy system and for optimum hair growth.

Q21 I am a twenty-five-year-old female and have recently noticed the hair on my face and body becoming thicker. I have also recently been diagnosed as suffering from female pattern baldness. Are these problems related? What should I do?

Normally, women who are genetically predisposed towards hair thinning notice the effects at menopause, but it's not impossible for symptoms to develop earlier. If a particular hormone imbalance (such as polycystic ovarian syndrome) is present, not only could your genetic hair thinning be induced, but an increase in the production of hair growth on your face and body may occur. You should request a blood test to check your hormone levels.

In cases such as yours, it would normally be of particular relevance to check your serum progesterone and serum testosterone levels together with your follicular stimulating hormone (FSH) and luteinizing hormone (LH) levels. FSH is secreted by the pituitary gland and controls the formation of eggs by the ovaries, LH is also secreted by the pituitary gland and controls the production of sex hormones by the ovaries. If an imbalance were to remain undiagnosed and subsequently untreated, both the hair thinning on the scalp and the increased hair growth on your face and body would needlessly progress further. Hence it's important to seek medical advice.

However, hirsutism (an increase in hair growth on the face and body) can occur without female androgenetic alopecia and is often due to familial tendencies; take a look at other females in your family. Hirsutism is frequently found among certain ethnic groups and in these cases hormonal imbalances are not to blame. Recommended management techniques of this condition are waxing, bleaching, shaving or electrolysis. Qualified trichologists often add hair removal techniques to their clinical services.

Q22 I am thirty-five and I have been diagnosed as suffering female pattern hair thinning. I still have a decent amount of hair and would like to look at any possible treatment methods that may help slow my hair loss and/or improve the quality of my existing hair growth. It seems that most hair treatments are only targeted at men. What is available for women?

Treatments for male hair loss certainly dominate the market (and the media). Women, however, do have treatments available to them, as follows:

Over-the-counter help: Minoxidil (Regaine) is the only product on sale over the counter that is a licensed hair loss treatment and can be used for female as well as male pattern hair loss (see Question 5).

The medical approach: medical practitioners usually recommend anti-androgen drugs for female androgenetic alopecia (these drugs aim to inhibit the action of androgens or male hormones). The contraceptive pill Dianette is often recommended. Dianette contains 2mg of the anti-androgen cyproterone acetate and if required this can temporarily be prescribed in higher doses of 50 or 100mg.

Spironolactone and flutamide are other medically recommended anti-androgen drugs. Spironolactone is most commonly used in the treatment of high blood pressure but it also acts as an anti-androgen.

However, before taking anti-androgen drugs, women will be advised by their doctor of all potential side-effects that could occur during use. These may include, for example, liver problems, weight changes and menstrual problems. So, *always seek medical advice before taking anti-androgen drugs.*

The Trichological Approach: under the direction of a qualified trichologist the use of topical (scalp applied) preparations may be used to reduce the effects of androgens (male hormones) on the hair. Other lifestyle factors will be examined, including the importance of plenty of protein and iron in the diet. This helps to improve hair follicle health whether hair loss is genetic or not (see Question 75 for corresponding food types).

Conditioning treatments to improve hair elasticity may also be administered as hair breakage alone creates a further loss in hair density; therefore, with the correct cosmetic treatment hair volume should increase.

In essence, the trichological approach will help ensure no other factors are to blame with your hair loss, together with appropriate advice and treatment given for the condition diagnosed.

Q23 How about hair transplants for women who suffer female pattern hair loss?

Recent developments in hair transplant techniques (see Question 11) have helped make hair surgery a viable option for some more severe cases of female pattern hair loss, but never before medical tests are performed to rule out any contributory underlying health issues. (Always seek qualified advice.)

In addition, the "donor site" would have to be in good health. If the hair intended for transplantation is very thin, then surgery is unwise. In these cases, special interwoven hairpieces (or wigs) are a better option. These are made to fit and are matched to the patient's hair colour and texture, giving a completely natural look.

See also Question 64: women, as well as men, can use cover-up sprays. These create the illusion of having thicker hair.

Q24 I tend to back-comb the hair around my crown area to give it a 'lift'; am I doing any harm?

In the short-term, no: the essential 'root lift' for a special occasion will cause no lasting damage. However, if this is part of your regular hairstyling routine then it could remove or damage the cuticle or outside layer of the hair shafts, leading to dull lifeless hair and ultimately hair breakage. See Question 26; learn how to minimise cuticle damage and take a look at the cuticle layer on the photograph showing the structure of a human hair.

Q25 Apart from having suffered some hair loss over the years, my hair is rather frizzy. I am currently using an anti-frizz shampoo and conditioner that work quite well but I feel I need something extra. What else could I use?

A hair serum would be a helpful addition to your current regime but would need to be applied carefully so that your hair doesn't end up looking flat, as this would allow greater exposure of any thinning areas (for the same reason, choose a product designed for fine hair). Serums are applied after shampooing and conditioning, after you have combed your hair through, and while it is still wet. A small amount should be used (about the size of a ten-pence piece), which should be rubbed into the palms of your hands and then worked into the middle lengths and ends of your hair, avoiding the hair growth nearest your scalp. Then style as usual.

Q26 I suffer with hereditary hair thinning. My hairdresser has suggested a hair colourant to add increased texture to my hair. Could this be harmful?

Go ahead! This is indeed a clever way of adding the illusion of increased body and texture to thin hair. Today's colouring techniques have come a long way, with fantastic results often achieved, but it is important to check that your hairdresser is an experienced colourist to ensure a careful, professional application.

Although changing the colour of your hair won't accelerate any underlying hair-thinning problem, some hair shaft damage is likely, particularly when lifting your hair colour to a lighter shade. During access to the important cortex layer of the hair shaft (where the desired change in hair colour is achieved), chemicals penetrate the cuticle layer causing a degree of destruction, (see the photograph below showing cuticle damage on a human hair). A damaged cuticle layer results in hair breakage, tangling and loss of shine. But all is not lost, there are ways to overcome this.

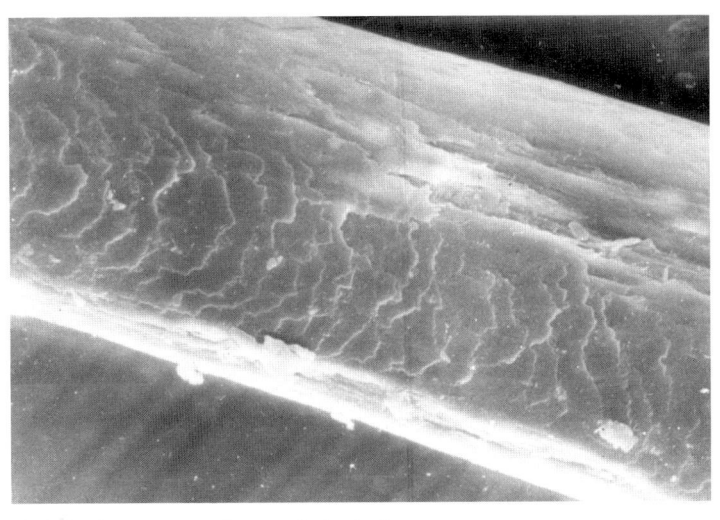

Cuticle damage on a human hair shaft
Photograph courtesy of Dr R. Dawber

Even if you have an excellent colourist, take a look at the following list of key points to remember when looking after your hair following chemical colouring.

Don't forget, poorly managed 'thin hair' will appear at least 20 per cent thinner than it really is.

Important key points to remember when looking after colour-treated hair:

   A To minimise cuticle damage always remember to apply a conditioning agent throughout the lengths of your hair after every shampoo and always leave the conditioner in contact with your hair for the time advised by the manufacturer (don't rush it), to ensure good results. These products smooth the cuticle layer to restore manageability and shine (for a healthy shampoo and conditioning technique see Question 65).

   B See Question 74; note the healthiest types of combs and brushes to use and never brush your hair when it is soaking wet – use a comb.

   C Always use the gentle de-tangling technique as explained on page 49 (part B).

   D Use a cooler (medium) heat setting on hairdryers and other heated styling aids.

   E When using hairdryers always maintain a distance of around fifteen inches between the machine and your hair during use.

   F Trim your hair every four to six weeks.

   G Always use fabric-covered hair bands or ties, not exposed elastic types.

   H When holidaying in sunny climates and while swimming in pools and the sea remember that chemically-treated hair will need extra protection against this potentially harmful combination of sun, chlorine and sea salt. Special sun protection products designed for hair are available through trichological practices and quality high street chemists in gel, spray and cream form. Most of these products protect against all of these 'holiday factors' and should also protect any areas of sun-exposed scalp.

Q27 I'm about to embark on my first 'hair colour experiment' but I have fairly sensitive skin. How could I check if I'm allergic to a hair colourant before I use it?

A 'patch' or 'sensitivity test' is recommended: smear a walnut-sized blob of the chosen colourant and a little activator to the skin of the scalp behind your ear and leave on for 24 to 48 hours. If you are sensitive or allergic to the agent, redness or sensitivity will appear on the specific area tested. Take this as a warning and do not use this product; ask the advice of your hairdresser or trichologist.

Alternatively, you may wish to opt for a salon routine whereby only specific sections of your hair are chemically treated while being wrapped in foil strips. This prevents the product coming into contact with your scalp.

Q28 Help! I am only twenty-two and my hair is definitely thinner than it used to be. Could this really be happening at such a young age and what could possibly be causing it?

Hair loss problems can strike at practically any age. The two checklists on the following pages should help.

1 Answer the following questions yes or no

A Are you noticing increased amounts of hair coming out when you shampoo, brush or comb your hair?
B Do you think your hair is thinner all over your scalp? Have you noticed that you can't fill your usual hair clips or ties as you used to?
C Have you recently experienced a sudden dramatic loss of weight?
D Have you suffered a very severe bout of stress recently?
E Have you been taking any prescribed medications over the last six to twelve months? (See page 21, where examples of some prescribed drugs that can cause hair loss are listed).

If you have answered yes to more than four points on this checklist your hair loss problem could be linked to health and lifestyle changes and/or stress. See pages 19–21; your type of hair loss falls into the non-pattern category, whereby increased hair shedding and an overall reduction in hair density is experienced, but you should make a full recovery.

Take these important steps now:

- request a blood test to find out, in particular, if you could be iron-deficient or if you have problems with an underactive or overactive thyroid gland;
- ensure you eat regularly during the day; don't skip meals and refer to Question 75 for the best 'hair foods'.

2 Answer the following questions yes or no

A Do you think that your hair is thinner on the top of your scalp as opposed to other areas?
B Have you noticed that your facial hair has increased or become darker in colour over recent years?
C Are you using any hormone-acting contraceptives at present or done so in the last six to twelve months?
D Is there a strong tendency towards hair thinning amongst the men and the women in your family?

If you have answered yes to at least three of the above points then it is possible that you have a genetic predisposition towards hair thinning. If you have answered yes to question B you need to be sure there are no underlying hormonal problems present, as these could exacerbate hereditary hair thinning or even mediate the problem if you are genetically predisposed.

Take these important steps now:

- request a blood test highlighting your serum progesterone and serum testosterone levels and both your FSH and LH levels. (See also Question 21);
- also check your iron levels and thyroid function;
- if you are using hormone-acting contraceptives, check with your doctor that you are not on any progestogen-only or high-strength combined formulas as they may accelerate the problem (see page 18).

PLEASE NOTE: This response is only a guide. For an accurate diagnosis you should consult a qualified trichologist. If blood tests are required the appropriate medical referrals will be made.

Q29 I'm a businesswoman who has to fly long haul frequently. Could this way of life be potentially harmful to my otherwise quite healthy hair?

Long haul flights are stressful on the body. Digestion, sleep patterns and even hormone production can all be temporarily disturbed. Where hair and frequent long haul flights are concerned, the hair growth cycle could be upset and acute telogen effluvium (see page 19) may develop.

Acute telogen effluvium results in an increase in the amount of hair reaching the resting stage of the hair growth cycle, resulting in an increase in hair shedding. This is a temporary problem but if you do experience some hair loss and your causative routine is unlikely to change, then hair re-growth could be slow.

Q30 Apart from other symptoms of premenstrual tension (PMT), I notice that my hair feels less lively and more drab just before my period is due. Why is this?

Oestrogen (the female hormone) levels are highest during the first half of the menstrual cycle and drop off during the second half – in the days leading up to a period. Oestrogen is in general a hair-positive hormone – for example, during pregnancy (when oestrogen dominates), women usually notice that their hair is in the best condition it has ever been. So we can point the finger of blame at these natural monthly hormone swings for bad hair days.

3

Children's Hair

Although hair problems, and in particular hair loss conditions, are generally uncommon in children, numerous questions are asked regarding children's hair. Some points are raised out of pure parental curiosity, while other questions in this chapter concern specific hair and scalp problems.

Q31 My children were born with quite a lot of hair. I know this isn't uncommon, but what I would love to know is when these 'first hairs' actually sprout.

Hair starts to grow by about the twentieth week of gestation. Such early development is said to afford the head some protection while inside the womb. This hair is called the 'lanugo' hair.

Q32 My baby is three months old. He's lost some hair from the middle of the back of his head. Is this anything to worry about?

This is termed 'occipital alopecia' and is not usually a cause for concern. The lanugo hair that develops in the womb enters the telogen or resting phase before birth, except for the hairs in the middle of the back of the head. These hairs enter the telogen phase between ten and twelve weeks after birth, temporarily leaving a visible bald area. However, by the time your baby is a year old, hair will be growing evenly all over the scalp.

Q33 My baby suffers with cradle cap. My GP has advised a weekly application of olive oil for an hour before shampooing, but it doesn't seem to be working. What else can I try which is both safe and effective?

Cradle cap is a term used to describe infantile seborrhoeic dermatitis/eczema, (see Question 61 for further information). A scalp effected by cradle cap is covered in a thick and often quite greasy layer of scale; this is why olive oil doesn't always help as it may just stick the scales together in an even thicker mass or will just penetrate the scales on the surface.

Firstly, never be afraid to shampoo your baby's hair/scalp every day as the scaling will only continue to build up. If this isn't enough by itself, then alternate between your usual brand of shampoo with one containing some de-scaling agents. Look out for a shampoo containing small quantities of coal tar (not above 1 per cent) and salicylic acid (not above 0.5 per cent) and dilute a ten pence piece sized blob with water (50/50 mix) before use. You may also find a couple of weekly applications of a gentle scalp cream designed for cradle cap very helpful in lifting the stubborn scale. If, however, the problem still persists seek the advice of a qualified trichologist.

It is also worth mentioning, while you are treating cradle cap, that you should resist the temptation to pick the scales off with your finger nails, combs or brushes. Such action could lead to a bacterial infection and permanent damage to your baby's scalp and hair. The best way to loosen the scaly build-up is to use gentle massage movements with the pads of your fingertips while shampooing and, if necessary, during the application of scalp treatment cream.

Q34 What sort of brush should I use on my one-year-old?

The younger the child, the smaller the brush; never use pointed or sharp bristles. Small, soft brushes specifically designed for babies can be bought in most pharmacies.

Q35 My child has repeatedly caught head lice during the last six months. How can I help prevent another infestation?

I am afraid there's no easy way to prevent your child from catching head lice, other than solitary confinement!

Head lice walk from one scalp to the next (they do not fly, as is often thought). Therefore, as children tend to play in close groups, head-to-head contact is almost inevitable. If you discover an infestation, inform your child's headteacher; an alert should also go out to other parents. It only takes a small number of untreated head lice cases in a school to increase the chances of constant re-infestation. For the same reason it is advised that you inform close friends and relatives as well, however antisocial this subject may seem.

During cycles of infestation, ensure your child wears

only their own hats, caps and hair bands and uses their own combs and brushes. Bedding and clothing need to be washed and dried using hot temperatures and brushes and combs should be washed on a daily basis in hot water.

Q36 I can't get rid of my daughter's head lice. I've treated her twice but she remains infested. What am I doing wrong?

There are two possible reasons why the problem persists. Firstly, are you using the lice medication properly? Ensure that you apply enough of the treatment to your daughter's head (one 'treatment' equals one whole allocated container of lotion or cream); don't be afraid to use it all and make sure you use it effectively. Apply it through small sections of hair at a time, reaching all around the scalp. Pouring it on one spot and 'spreading it all around' isn't good enough (see

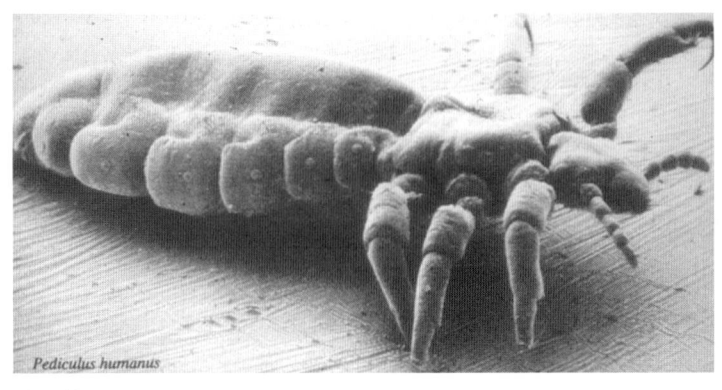

Head louse
Photograph courtesy of Dr R. Dawber

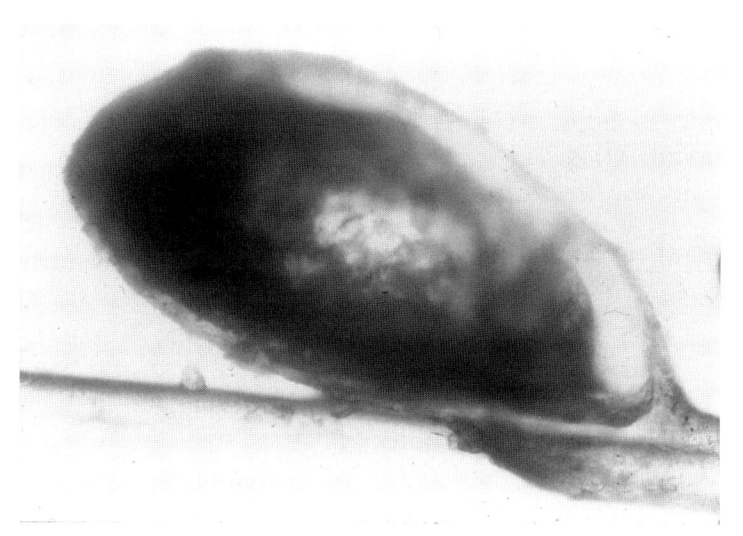

Louse egg/nit attached to a hair shaft
Photograph courtesy of Dr R. Dawber

Question 38 where some recommended lice treatments are listed; always ensure you study the manufacturer's instructions carefully before use).

Secondly, as part of the treatment procedure, are you removing all of the lice eggs (or nits)? Any 'live' nits left behind will hatch very quickly (see Question 37). It is therefore imperative to ensure that all nits have been removed following the use of lice treatment. Initially the eggs are quite difficult to detect and remove, but with perseverance the task becomes easier. The eggs are oval in shape and often yellow when freshly laid (as opposed to grey/white when hatched) (see the photograph above). You'll find them wrapped tightly around the hair shafts, most predominately around the ears and across the back of neck.

For efficient nit removal, use a special nit detection

comb (available at any pharmacy). Dampen the hair down a little (use a water-filled spray bottle), because you will be combing it many times and parting it off into sections, which is a little easier when the hair is damp. Make sure that you work on small sections of hair at a time. Catch the eggs between the teeth of the comb and then ease them down towards the ends of the hair shafts. This is a time-consuming procedure, but worth the extra effort.

PLEASE NOTE: Your daughter should not use hair-dryers or other heat-emitting hairstyling equipment during the administration of lice treatment as the heat produced from these machines retards the effects of the chemicals applied.

Q37 How long does it take for a lice egg to hatch?

Only seven to ten days I'm afraid, which is why it's imperative to treat these infestations as quickly as possible!

Q38 What are the best anti-lice products on the market?

I receive positive feedback from parents who have used products that contain either permethrin or phenothrin as the main active ingredient. Application times are shorter with these chemicals and phenothrin can be administered in the form of a mousse. This has the advantage that it is difficult to miss a patch when your child's head is covered in foam! Also, I suspect young children find this sort of treatment 'fun' and they may cooperate better during an application as a result.

These products are available over the counter, but if you have a really stubborn case of head lice, your doctor can prescribe a product containing carbaryl. One treatment, or application, of an agent containing carbaryl should be enough to clear an infestation.

Q39 When is it safe to use conditioner on my child's hair? Should I wait until she is a certain age?

It is quite safe to use conditioner on your daughter's hair at any time during her development, particularly if her hair is long (e.g. below the earlobes). It is always advised that you apply conditioner from the middle to the tips of the hair lengths for best results (see Question 65).

Q40 My son is eight years old and has suddenly developed a bald patch. I've heard of alopecia in adults; is it possible in children? And how about 'ringworm'? I've been told this can cause hair loss.

Specialised tests should be carried out to formally diagnose a case of ringworm (a fungal infection). Trichologists use a 'Wood's Lamp'; an ultraviolet light that shows clearly the presence of ringworm. If this test proves positive your trichologist will refer your child to your GP for administration of anti-fungal agents.

As a general guide however, the difference between

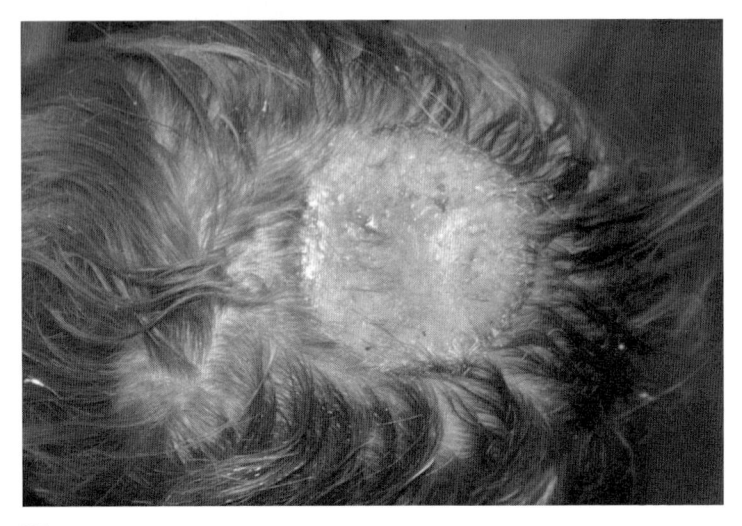

Ringworm
Photograph courtesy of Dr R. Dawber

alopecia areata (patchy hair loss) and ringworm is that the scalp usually appears beautifully clear and healthy in the case of alopecia areata, but scaling and pus production is evident with ringworm (alopecia areata is discussed further in Question 69). In either case, you'll need to refer to your trichologist or GP.

Q41 My ten-year-old daughter has very long hair that she loves to wear loose, but on a daily basis she complains about terrible tangling, especially of the hair around her collar area. How can this be avoided?

Make sure that she always applies a conditioner to her hair after shampooing (this should be left on for at least five minutes). After conditioning, she needs to squeeze any excess water from her hair and lightly pat dry with a towel. This should be followed by some gentle de-tangling (see page 49, part B, for advice on the ideal de-tangling technique). At this stage she could spray on a light de-tangling product; these help ease de-tangling and they introduce a 'fun' incentive to this otherwise rather boring procedure.

Finally she must ensure that she thoroughly dries her hair. The hair at the collar (or nape area) is often neglected, as it is a difficult area to reach while drying/styling especially if a person has a lot of long hair to cope with. If (in particular) the hair at the nape area remains damp it will dry 'crinkled', allowing it to tangle even more easily. Your daughter needs to direct a hairdryer on a medium heat setting towards this difficult section of hair while gently teasing it straight.

Alternatively, she should consider the idea of tying her hair back (at least on school days), although she must always use soft fabric-covered ties and not uncovered or exposed elastic bands, as these cause hair breakage.

Q42 I have just turned twelve years old. By my thirteenth birthday I want my hair to be past my shoulders (it is just above them at the moment). I realise I will still need to trim my hair to keep it in good condition but how often and how much should I cut off each time to finally obtain my goal of long, healthy hair?

Hair grows at a rate of half an inch a month. A trim of half an inch every two months will remove unhealthy split ends. By this reckoning, three inches of good conditioned hair can be grown in a year. See also Question 87.

Q43 My son is only thirteen years old and I have noticed that his hairline has receded slightly. Is this cause for concern?

At puberty, slight hairline recession is very common among boys and girls. Don't panic, he's not about to lose all of his hair and this doesn't necessarily mean that he will go on to develop male pattern baldness in later years.

Q44 My daughter has just hit puberty and I have noticed that her hair and scalp is starting to smell badly even though she shampoos three times a week. Why is this happening and how can we treat it?

This is usually due to the hormonal changes that occur at this stage. At this time of life, sebaceous glands, responsible for the production of scalp oil (sebum), begin producing stronger, potentially smelly oil. It is advised that she starts shampooing her hair daily. If she uses conditioner ensure she only applies it to her hair and not to her scalp (this could make a greasy problem worse). However, of course, a conditioner should leave a pleasant perfume behind on her hair, which could prove helpful under these circumstances. Also, check that her diet is not too rich in spicy foods or fatty dairy produce. If the problem persists, consult your doctor.

4
Afro-Caribbean Hair

Afro-Caribbean hair is by nature extremely difficult to manage and style because it is so very tightly curled. Most trichological problems found with Afro-Caribbean hair are commonly linked to the procedures that are used to improve its manageability, as discussed below.

Chemical relaxing

Chemical relaxing involves the application of a product that contains a chemical (usually sodium hydroxide) that can permanently relax or straighten curly hair; sodium hydroxide and its alternatives are highlighted under Question 49.

However, problems arise if sloppy techniques are employed. Damage occurs when a chemical relaxer is left in contact with the hair longer than is necessary or technically recommended (a common problem during the self-application of home relaxer kits). Problems also develop if a chemical relaxer is applied to hair that has already been chemically treated, or if the relaxing procedure is carried out too often, such as every three or four weeks, instead of the recommended ideal frequency of eight to twelve weeks. See page 50 (part F) and Questions 45 and 46.

Hot comb pressing

Hot comb pressing is a non-chemical straightening procedure and involves a heated comb being passed through the hair repeatedly until it straightens. The heat applied needs to be very high indeed and although it is an aggressive procedure the effects of straightening are only temporary. If the hair gets wet it will revert back to its original texture again, resulting in such frequent use that hair and scalp damage is almost inevitable.

Hair extensions

Although Afro-Caribbean hair grows at the usual rate (see Question 42) it seems to take a lot longer because it's so tightly curled. Therefore, hair extensions are often used to create some useful extra length in an instant.

However, problems arise when extensions are fitted too tightly and repeatedly left in longer than around eight weeks at a time; they can pull the hair out of the scalp (worst case scenario), gradually weaken hair growth and can even eventually cause localised, painful scalp disorders.

Braiding

Braiding is another hairstyling option and is commonly adopted by children as well as adults. However, braids worn too tightly, or left in for too long, can cause 'traction' hair loss along the front hairline as well as in between each braid. In particular, if such trauma is continually applied to children's hair it may, in time, become irreversibly weak, ultimately leading to a reduced hair growth potential in adulthood. See page

50 (part G) for tips on healthy braiding. Traction alopecia is discussed further in Question 47.

However, all is not lost. There's a lot that can be done to prevent short- and long-term damage. For the preservation of a full and healthy head of Afro-Caribbean hair and a clear and healthy scalp, observe the following guidelines.

Important key points to remember when looking after Afro-Caribbean hair

A Keep up maintenance techniques such as conditioning/steaming treatments. Steaming is very useful as Afro-Caribbean hair absorbs moisture easily which in turn helps improve its elasticity.

B Always handle your hair with the greatest of care. For instance, while de-tangling always use a wide-toothed comb. Work on small sections of hair at a time, starting from the ends of the hair lengths, gradually working your way up towards the scalp area. Never pass a comb (or brush) straight from your scalp to the tips of your hair lengths in one hit until all the knots have been removed; this type of aggressive handling can cause hair breakage. See Questions 73 and 74; find out when it is best to brush or comb (when your hair is wet or dry), and learn which types of combs and brushes are healthiest.

C Avoid wearing hair curlers in bed at night. This can cause hair breakage and may eventually pull the hair out from the scalp. On the subject of hair curlers, in particular, do not use self-gripping (or velcro/brush) rollers. These can potentially damage the outer cuticle layer of the hair shafts causing extensive hair breakage.

D It pays to use shampoos, conditioners and hair creams/greases specifically for Afro-Caribbean hair. Trichologists prepare these for individual requirements.

E Never massage leave-on hair conditioners or grease into a sensitive scalp; use these through the lengths of your *hair* only. This attention to detail avoids a build-up on your scalp, which may lead to irritation or soreness, especially as you may only shampoo weekly or fortnightly. If your scalp requires moisturising then apply aqueous cream to your scalp instead (see Questions 45 and 52).

F When chemically relaxing fine-textured Afro-Caribbean hair, the chemical should only be in contact for up to a maximum of three minutes (as opposed to the four to seven minutes required to chemically relax medium to thick hair types).

G Avoid wearing braids for more than two weeks at a time; take a week off between resuming this hairstyle for another fortnight and braid thicker sections of hair to reduce tension at scalp level.

Women should also refer to Question 26 (pages 32–33) under the section entitled Important key points to remember when looking after colour-treated hair.

The following questions are frequently encountered regarding Afro-Caribbean hair.

Q45 Due to long-term exposure to chemical relaxers and a succession of subsequent minor chemical burns, my scalp remains extremely sensitive even though I was successfully treated following these incidences. In particular, moisturising products really irritate my scalp. Which ingredient in these products could be to blame?

It's difficult to pin point an exact culprit, but lanolin, coconut oil and almond oil could be potentially irritating, especially if you have an extremely sensitive scalp. Of course, the problem here is that most Afro-Caribbean moisturising or grease-based hair products contain these ingredients. So it's down to careful application, taking care to apply these products to your hair only and apply moisture-giving aqueous cream (a non-irritant water-based emollient) on your scalp instead. Aqueous cream is also mentioned under Question 52 and is available through high street chemists.

If this 'self-help' doesn't work for you, consultant a qualified trichologist.

Q46 I chemically relax my hair every four weeks but it's starting to break, particularly at the back of my neck. Could this be linked to the chemicals and, if so, what can I do about it?

Chemical relaxing can indeed cause hair breakage particularly if it is carried out with such regularity and especially if this has been part of your hairstyling routine for a long time. The nape area (at the back of your neck) is particularly vulnerable as the relaxer is often applied here first during processing; therefore this section of hair growth is exposed to the effects of the chemical agents longer than the rest of your hair.

Reduce chemical processing to every eight to twelve weeks and when re-touching re-growth always check during application that the relaxing product is not overlapping onto your previously relaxed hair. Always ensure that chemical relaxers are never left on longer than ten minutes.

Resist using aggressive blow-drying and styling techniques and do not apply excessively high temperatures to your hair. All of these can encourage hair breakage in any case, let alone if your hair is already chemically processed.

It is also advised that you regularly trim and steam your hair.

Q47 I am a healthy black female without any history of balding in my family, but my front hairline is receding (including the areas around my ears) and a noticeable amount of general hair breakage is occurring. What could be causing this?

This type of hair loss is generally termed traumatic cosmetic alopecia, although your situation is often further classified as traction alopecia (see the photograph on the following page). As the term suggests, it describes hair loss caused by the effects of persistent traumatic forces (such as pulling or dragging) being applied to the hair. It often affects the front hairline but it can occur anywhere that constant tension is applied; braiding is a common cause as are hair extensions, tightly-worn ponytails and vigorous hair-straightening procedures.

Trace your steps. Have you worn your hair in any of these styles or employed techniques such as hot comb

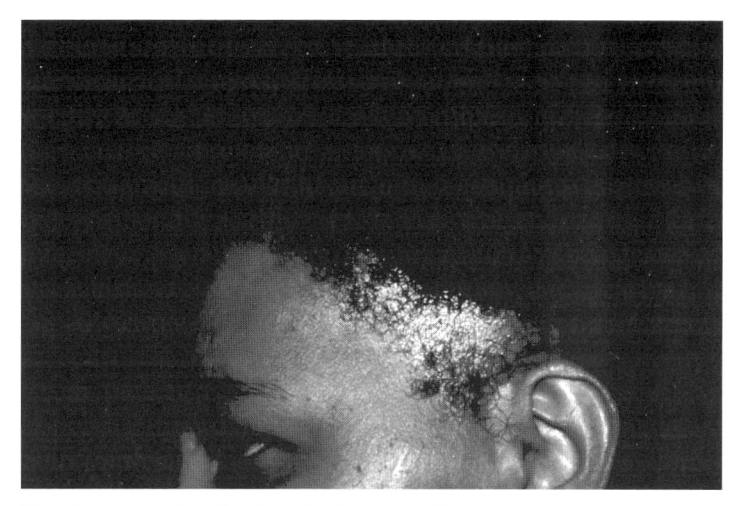

Traction alopecia affecting the front hairline
Photograph courtesy of Dr R. Dawber

pressing for long periods of time? Try to vary the way you wear your hair to reduce such trauma. If the causative factors are removed (and as long as no permanent damage has occurred to the hair follicles), your hair will have a chance to strengthen again.

Q48 I have been told since childhood that hair extensions can make your hair grow faster, but I have also heard that they can actually pull your hair out; what is the truth?

It is biologically impossible for hair extensions to make your hair grow faster. Regarding 'pulling your hair out': if extensions are attached so tight they cause you pain and your scalp becomes tender to touch, then hair loss could easily occur. As highlighted on page 48 under

'Hair Extensions', don't leave them in longer than eight weeks at a time – this applies even if the extensions have been fitted correctly without excessive tension.

Q49 Are 'no lye relaxers' safer than standard products?

Frankly, there is no such thing as a safe chemical relaxer. 'No lye relaxers' are products that do not contain aggressive sodium hydroxide but do contain either potassium, calcium or lithium hydroxide instead. These chemicals act on the hair in much the same way as sodium hydroxide and could therefore be as potentially harmful. However, the UK has recently seen more widespread use of guanidine hydroxide relaxers. Although guanidine hydroxide is still a chemical, it is considered milder than other no lye relaxers. However, as with all chemicals, care should always be taken during use.

Q50 I have always kept my hair in its natural state, but now I would like to chemically relax it occasionally. Would a guanidine relaxer be a better option for someone like me who isn't accustomed to using chemicals?

A guanidine relaxer would be a less aggressive option for you, especially as you're a newcomer to chemical relaxing. However, always exercise caution during application and take into account all the possible pitfalls commonly associated with chemical relaxing now to avoid any future problems. See page 47 and Questions 45 and 46, where all these possible negative factors are highlighted.

Q51 I've been braiding my hair to give it a break from chemical relaxing. Unfortunately, I haven't spent as much time and effort on conditioning regimes as I originally intended, and now I would like to chemically relax my hair again. Are there any important guidelines to follow before going back to chemicals?

When you take your braids out, don't use any chemicals for at least a fortnight. During this period, undertake some intensive conditioning treatments to ensure that your hair is up to the chemical challenge again (a trichologist would devise a treatment plan for you). Remember a reputable hairdresser will only apply chemicals to your hair if they feel it is strong enough; always make sure you're in good hands.

Q52 I am a healthy male without any past history of skin problems, but in recent months I've begun suffering with spots or 'bumps' on the back of my neck. These irritate and bleed. Just before these eruptions appeared I started using clippers and razors as I wanted to keep my hair really short; could there be any connection?

Clippers or razors are capable of causing scalp and skin problems. If they are not thoroughly sterilised before use, or if they damage your skin while you are using them, then hair follicles may become infected. This condition is called folliculitis nuchae. Due to the irritation generated by this problem, and the subsequent scratching of the scalp, the infection is spread quickly and it can cause permanent hair loss if left untreated.

Seek the help of a qualified trichologist; this condition is usually treated effectively by topical antibacterial agents. However, it is essential that during the administration of any scalp treatment you must resist the use of any hair clippers or razors, as there is every chance that they will knock the healing 'protrusions' making them bleed and thus spreading the infection even further. Get your barber to use their scissors instead; it is also advised that you maintain the use of scissors instead of clippers and razors even once the infection has cleared, to prevent folliculitis nuchae occuring again.

If you usually use a scalp moisturising agent then it's advised you use simple aqueous cream instead of your usual product, in case this worsens the irritation (see Question 45).

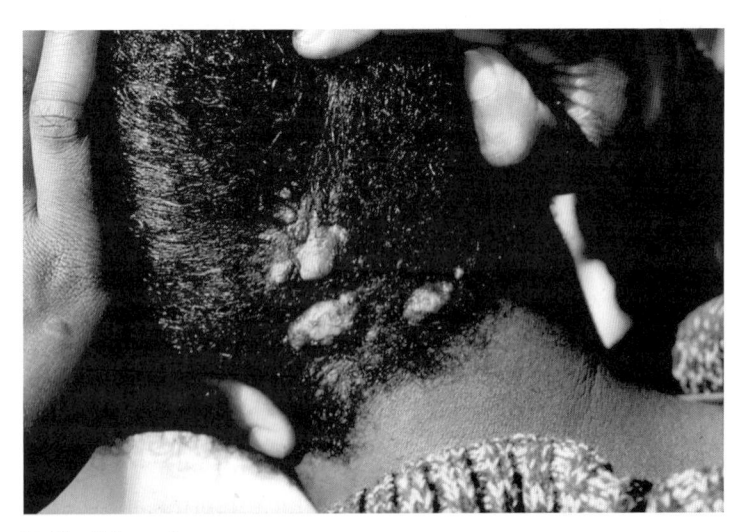

Folliculitis nuchae
Photograph courtesy of Dr R. Dawber

5

General Hair and Scalp Facts

The following questions and answers highlight a myriad of issues that involve both the scalp and the hair.

Q53 Can regular physical exercise increase or decrease hair loss?

The only time exercise could be a reason for exacerbated hair loss is when performance-enhancing drugs are taken as part of the regime (not the sort of activity a normal person would pursue), or when an individual 'overdoes it' on a regular basis, such as exercise junkies.

On the positive side, all our body systems benefit from a regular, sensible exercise routine, therefore general hair health could be given a boost too – but not in a corrective sense; exercise doesn't decrease hair loss.

Q54 Could regular scalp massage promote hair growth?

Scalp massage performed alone (without the application of any topical or scalp-applied hair loss treatment; see Questions 5 and 22) doesn't promote hair growth.

However, a therapeutic effect is achieved by improving blood circulation, encouraging the removal of waste products from the scalp and reducing muscle tension (very useful, especially with the impossible-to-exercise scalp area), and it is of course very relaxing. These effects boost hair health, improving its vitality and helping to reduce scalp pain or tenderness. Gentle scalp massage is also recommended for women in the early days of the menopause, as this is a time when the scalp can feel unusually tight and sometimes tender.

Check your massage technique: while using the pads of your fingertips, gently move the scalp over the skull. Do not let your fingertips vigorously rub the scalp in any way. I have met individuals who believed excessive rubbing of the scalp was beneficial to hair growth – until their hair broke off at scalp level.

Q55 Is it true that hair grows at a faster rate in the summer?

Yes. More sunlight and warmer temperatures increase the rate of cell division in hair follicles, producing a slight increase in the rate of hair growth. However, hair (and any exposed areas of scalp) will need protection against strong sunlight; take a look at Questions 3 and 26 (part H).

Q56 Why do I see more hair come out when I haven't shampooed for two or three days as opposed to when I shampoo daily?

On a daily basis up to a hundred hairs are naturally shed from the scalp, having come to the end of the anagen or active growth phase; see page 22 under 'The hair growth cycle'). Under normal circumstances these hairs are replaced without us noticing a reduction in hair quantity. During the action of shampooing (and combing and brushing), most of these hairs are naturally discarded.

Therefore, if you do not shampoo your hair for two or three days then two to three days' worth (or up to two to three hundred) of these telogen hairs will have accumulated, ready for you to see collected at the bottom of the shower.

Q57 I am a regular swimmer. Could the chlorine in my local swimming baths damage my hair or accelerate my hair loss problem?

Chlorine tends to react with the cuticle or outside protective layer of the hair shaft, and any negative reaction against the cuticle layer results in dull, unmanageable hair (see Question 26). It has also been found that copper ions from swimming pools can leave a green tinge to naturally blonde or bleached hair, but these negative effects on the hair shafts alone would not cause hair loss or accelerate an existing hair thinning problem.

It is advised that you thoroughly shampoo and condition your hair after every swim. Check that your favourite shampoo contains a reducing agent such as sodium thiosulfate to ensure the chlorine is easily removed from the hair (reducing the risk of cuticle damage). Also included should be a chelating agent such as tetrasodium EDTA or trisodium thiosulfate, to clear any copper residues from the hair and to prevent (and remove) any green discoloration problems.

If in doubt about the contents of your shampoo, check it with a qualified trichologist. There are products available that are made for frequent swimmers and contain all the necessary ingredients. A trichologist will advise on a product that will suit both your hair and your sports routine.

Q58 I suffer with dandruff. Are there any particular foods I should be avoiding?

It has been suspected that spicy foods, full fat milk, cheeses, lager and red wines may aggravate dandruff (and seborrhoeic dermatitis). Although this might not be the case for every sufferer, you could try a fortnight without these foods and drinks and then introduce them again one by one to see which (if any) triggers a return of dandruff. See Question 61 for information on the causes of dandruff and seborrhoeic dermatitis.

Q59 I pull my own hair out. It is a terrible habit and results in visible bald patches. I am in a desperate state. How can I stop it?

This is a condition called trichotillomania; and commonly follows a traumatic experience or a prolonged period of stress. Once the habit takes hold it can be very difficult (but certainly not impossible) to break. The best thing to do is keep a diary for a week and record when you most often attempt to pull your hair out. Most sufferers find it happens when they are at rest, such as watching the television, on the telephone or when reading. Once you have found a pattern to this behaviour, you can set yourself certain tasks to

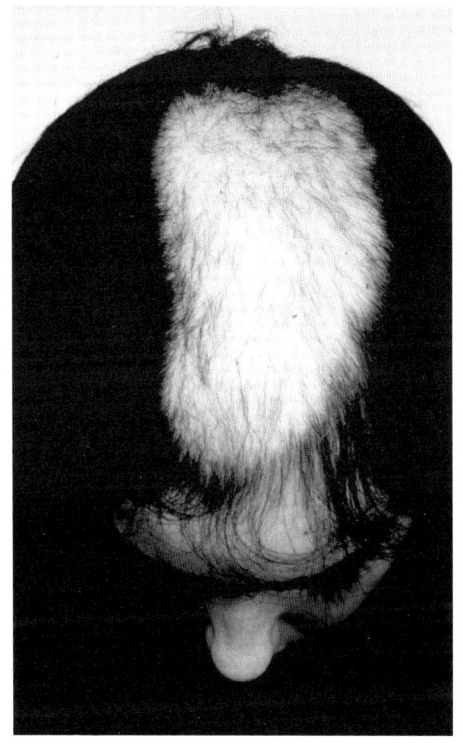

Trichotillomania
Photograph courtesy of Dr R. Dawber

keep your hands away from your scalp (knitting, drawing or sewing for example). I once had a client who wore a pair of mittens around the house when she returned home from work!

If this self-help technique does not work for you, then some form of counselling could be helpful. I have met trichotillomania sufferers who have successfully used psychologists and even hypnotists. Happily, in most cases once the habit is broken, hair will re-grow normally and quickly. Only when the follicles have been permanently damaged will hair re-growth be impossible.

Q60 I am due a course of chemotherapy, what do you think will happen to my hair?

Chemotherapy targets and attacks all actively dividing cells in the body whether they are healthy or not. Good news where cancerous tumours are concerned but disastrous for the continually dividing cells of hair follicles. A temporary halt in activity is therefore likely, although not entirely definite as it depends on the dose and type of drug(s) used; further advice can be obtained from your oncologist.

If you do suffer hair loss, it may become apparent within the early days of treatment, but the first signs of hair re-growth are usually noticed between four and six weeks after the course of treatment has finished (sometimes earlier). Happily, many people notice their new hair growth is actually healthier than before the chemotherapy was administered. However, if you are used to colouring or bleaching your hair, wait at least six months before doing so again.

If you manage to keep most (or all) of your hair during treatment, then be sure to handle it carefully – you may find that it will be quite dry and brittle. Avoid hairdryers or other heat-emitting styling aids and do not vigorously brush your hair. The gentle use of a wide-toothed comb is a better alternative, especially if you have long hair.

PLEASE NOTE: 'Cold caps' can be worn during the administration of chemotherapy. By freezing hair follicles, the cell division rate will be slowed down. This deceives the drug(s) into thinking that cell division does not take place and will therefore leave them alone. Cold caps aren't in regular hospital use as yet, and their efficiency is far from guaranteed, but it's definitely worth asking your oncologist whether your hospital provides them.

Q61 I have recently been diagnosed as suffering from seborrhoeic dermatitis. I thought I only suffered from dandruff. What's the difference?

These two common scalp complaints are linked by the same causes; in fact seborrhoeic dermatitis is often classified as a severe form of dandruff. Genetic factors

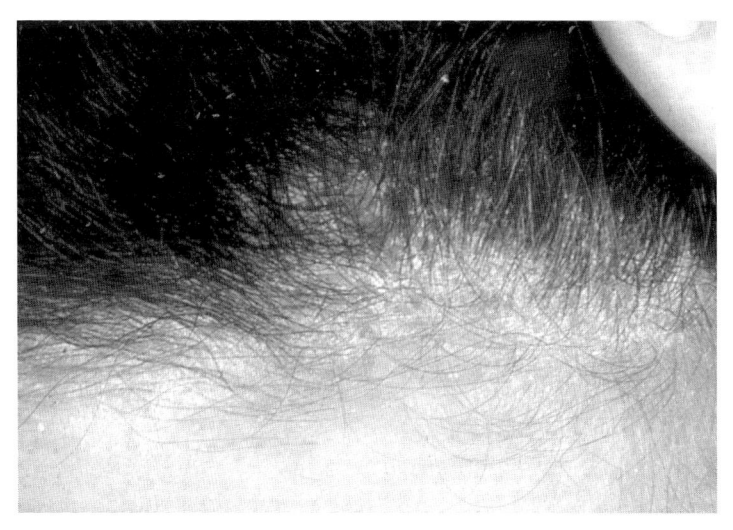

Seborrhoeic dermatitis
Photograph courtesy of Dr R. Dawber

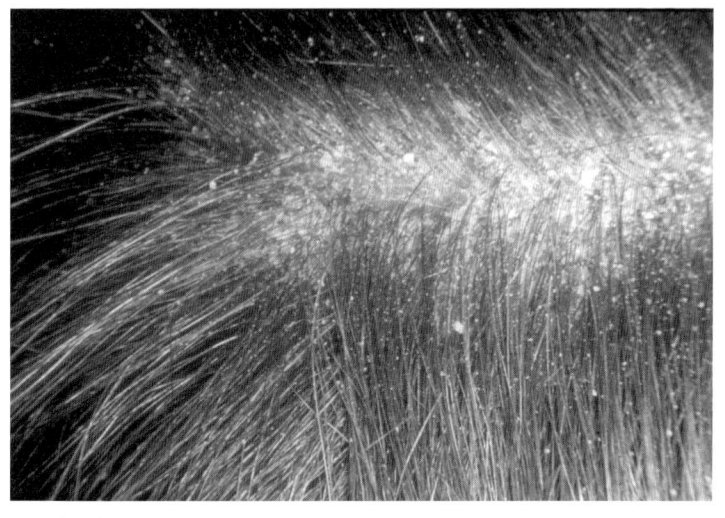

Dandruff
Photograph courtesy of Dr R. Dawber

play a part in both conditions, although they do not appear until puberty; increased sebum (oil) production, an inclination towards increased cell turnover from the epidermis (upper section of the skin) and the presence of the fungi pityrosporum ovale are all to blame. However, pityrosporum ovale is found in far greater quantities with seborrhoeic dermatitis than dandruff.

The main differences between seborrhoeic dematitis and dandruff are threefold: appearance, 'irritation factor', and location (on the body). Scalp redness, heavy scaling and intense itchiness is associated with seborrhoeic dermatitis; dandruff presents itself with some minor inflammation that is only visible under close examination under magnification and this is not usually obvious to the sufferer. Dandruff does not irritate and is associated only with the appearance of small, white scales. Seborrhoeic dermatitis appears not only on the scalp but also on the forehead, in the eyebrows, around the folds of the nose, around the groin and along the centre of the back and chest. Dandruff *only* affects the scalp. In comparison to seborrhoeic dermatitis, dandruff is purely a cosmetic hindrance.

Babies who suffer with cradle cap (a heavy scale covering the scalp) often go on to develop seborrhoeic dermatitis in their teens (cradle cap is discussed in Question 33).

Whether you suffer with seborrhoeic dermatitis or ordinary dandruff, always shampoo daily, do not apply conditioners to your scalp, do not massage gels and mousses into your scalp and avoid using 2 in 1 products (shampoos pre-mixed with a conditioner).

The food types that may aggravate dandruff could also aggravate seborrhoeic dermatitis; these are listed under Question 58.

With the correct guidance, seborrhoeic dermatitis is easy to manage. A qualified trichologist will provide specific treatments that retard skin cell turnover as well as reducing the presence of pityrosporum ovale and other fungi (without the use of heavy-duty chemicals) to maintain a healthy scalp that's free from scaliness and irritation.

Dandruff control is discussed in Question 68.

Q62 I suffer with psoriasis on my scalp. Could this prevent normal, healthy hair growth?

Psoriasis usually forms in patches over the scalp and unfortunately in the worst affected areas, hair growth can be impaired. The hair shafts often break off close

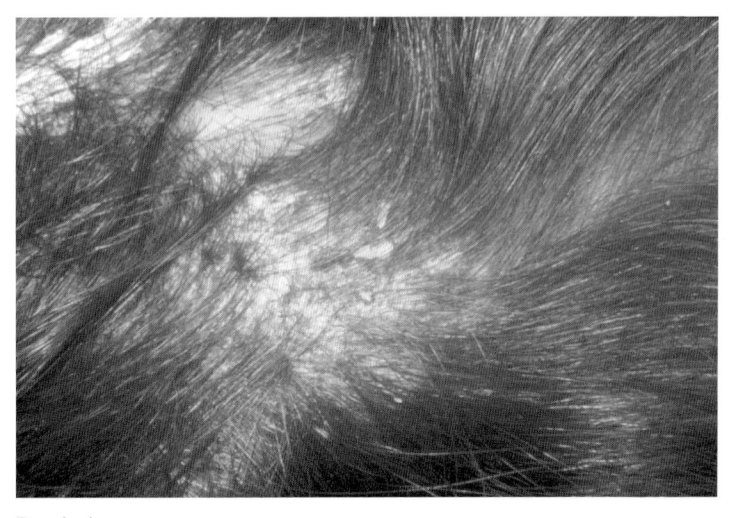

Psoriasis
Photograph courtesy of Dr R. Dawber

to the scalp and in extreme, chronic cases of scalp psoriasis hair can become thinner or weaker due to hair follicle atrophy (wasting). However, if psoriasis is successfully managed, hair growth reacts positively too.

Psoriasis is predominately a genetic condition, therefore the aim is to control it, not cure it. It seems that the skin cell turnover rate in the epidermis (upper section of the skin) is five times faster than in non-psoriatic skin. Normally, a cell takes four to six weeks to reach the surface of the skin (from where it is removed); with psoriasis sufferers, this process only takes around nine days, which explains the continuous build-up of scaly scab formations.

Stress has long been thought of as a contributing factor to this problem, as have systemic infections and hormonal problems. Foods such as dairy products, tomatoes, seafood products, diluted orange juice and alcohol could aggravate psoriasis as well.

It is advised that you seek the advice of a qualified trichologist where scalp psoriasis is concerned. Depending on the individual case, trichologists formulate shampoos, scalp solutions and creams that both remove the scaly build-up and retard its re-formation. Ultraviolet light therapy is also employed by trichologists when treating psoriasis.

Q63 I have been prescribed some steroid cream for a persistent scalp problem. Can steroids cause hair thinning?

Steriods can cause skin to thin if used for many years. If you're planning to use steroids on the scalp continuously, then eventually you may find that your hair could be adversely affected where the cream is most frequently applied. Nowadays, most medical practitioners rarely suggest such long-term use of topical steroids.

Trichologists formulate products that can be used on a regular basis without generating any such side-effects. Seek the advice of a qualified trichologist; they will steer you down a non-steroid path, along with introducing some diet modifications if appropriate.

Q64 I have a scar on my head from a childhood injury. It's completely bald! I would like to cover it up – any ideas?

If the scarred area is quite small (up to three inches in diameter), then hair mascaras are excellent (they can be found in hair salons or larger department stores). Designed to place temporary streaks of colour through hair, they are safe to wear directly on the scalp. Good quality hair mascaras are hard-wearing in wet weather and come in many colours.

Along similar lines are cover-up sprays that temporarily colour the exposed scalp to match your hair. These products are most commonly used by individuals suffering male or female pattern baldness (or androgenetic alopecia), but would also be ideal in your situation. Cover-up sprays are available in high street chemists or by mail order. Also, hair transplant surgery is becoming increasingly successful in relocating hair into scar tissue.

If you have a large bald area then an individually-designed hairpiece could be worn; this is attached to the scarred area with special adhesives (secure even during sports activities). Refer to page 7 (Question 5); the hair used is either human or synthetic, but either way it would be made to look natural. Always seek the advice of a trichologist, who (depending on the size and nature of your scarred area) will help you find a good cover-up product or put you in contact with a reputable hairpiece specialist or hair transplant surgeon.

Q65 I am not sure whether I shampoo my hair properly. Can you advise on the best technique?

Here is a step-by-step guide:
  A Always wet your hair thoroughly before the application of shampoo. Shampoos work best on saturated hair. Ensure that you rinse well; any

shampoo that gets left behind will make your hair look extremely dull.

B While shampooing long hair, always keep it flowing backwards in the direction of hair growth, not against it. This avoids excessive tangling. For example, avoid shampooing your hair with your head leaning over the side of the bath; shampoo under the shower instead.

C When applying shampoo, do not pour it straight from the bottle onto your head. Put some in the palm of your hand, rub your palms together for a second then spread it evenly over your scalp.

D Massage the shampoo into your scalp; do not scrub it through the lengths of your hair. During the rinsing process shampoo will pass through the lengths, cleaning them thoroughly.

E Do not dig your nails into your scalp; massage the shampoo into your scalp with the pads of your fingertips using gentle circular movements, working from the front hairline all the way back to the nape (back of neck) area.

F Shampoo once if you wash your hair every day, but two washes are best if you shampoo less than this.

G Before applying conditioner, squeeze any excess water out of your hair. Take hold of your conditioner and follow point C all over again, but do not massage the conditioner into your scalp. Work the conditioner through the lengths of your hair with your fingers; do not comb it through. Finally, ensure you rinse the conditioner out of your hair thoroughly.

Q66 I can 'pick' the odd strand of hair off my clothes quite frequently during the day. I have never heard my work colleagues or my friends complain of this with their hair, but I have always worn my hair very long, (waist length); could this be a problem?

Hair will enter a normal daily cycle of shedding (and replacement) as mentioned in other answers (see in particular page 22 where the hair growth cycle is explained). It is possible to shed about a hundred hairs on a daily basis. Although wearing your hair long will not make it fall out, it is far easier to notice long rather than short hair strands stuck to your clothes (and hairbrush) on a day-to-day basis.

How often do you shampoo? Most people with very long hair only shampoo about once a week, and this could be another reason why you notice dead hairs (as opposed to your colleagues and friends who may wear their hair shorter and are therefore likely to shampoo more often). See Question 56 for more information.

I notice that you do not mention anything about your hair feeling progressively thinner – check to see if you can still 'fill-up' your usual hair ties: do they fall off? Do you need to tighten them further than you did a year ago?

If you always wear your hair 'down' and, just 'feel' a general overall loss of hair density, then you may indeed have a trichological problem that needs some help.

Q67 My beard has bald patches. Are they likely to recover?

As long as the hair follicles remain intact, then hair regrowth is possible. Be patient, alopecia areata (a common form of patchy hair loss) of the beard can be particularly slow in healing. I advise a visit to a qualified trichologist to confirm alopecia areata, and not another form of hair loss that could be permanent. For example, severe forms of facial acne can cause hair loss in a 'patchy' formation, especially in the beard region; however, due to scarring the hair would be unable to grow back in these cases (see also Question 69).

Q68 Is it safe to use anti-dandruff shampoos all of the time?

If you feel the need to use anti-dandruff shampoos so frequently, perhaps you don't have dandruff at all. You could be suffering from a condition a little more severe, such as seborrhoeic dermatitis (see Question 61), or even psoriasis (see Question 62). Check this with a qualified trichologist immediately.

Simple cases of dandruff are normally successfully controlled with daily shampooing, using an anti-dandruff shampoo and a regular 'non-treatment' shampoo on an alternate basis.

Q69 I am twenty-five years old and since my late teens I have suffered two bouts of alopecia areata (patchy hair loss). My hair grew back each time but it did leave me wondering why it had occurred. My friends tell me it's a stress-linked condition but I don't think that I'm a stressed person, so what is the cause?

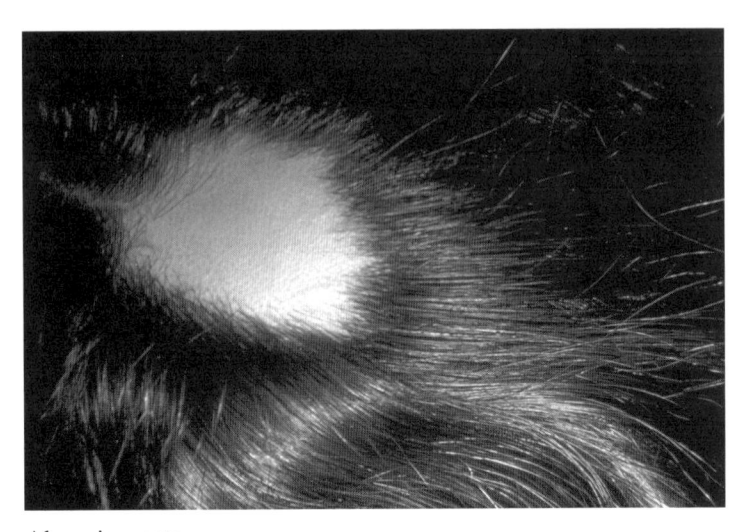

Alopecia areata
Photograph courtesy of Dr R. Dawber

To date, it is still very difficult to pinpoint what exactly causes alopecia areata. The most common point of view is that due to possible underlying hereditary factors the autoimmune system does not recognise the body's own 'self' components and will attack healthy hair follicle cells as it would an invading bacteria or virus.

Of course, stress doesn't help and it is possible to be suffering from stress and not know it. In fact it may well be a contributing factor. I've met many alopecia areata sufferers who have found particular relaxation techniques (e.g. regular exercise and yoga) of great help. Such activities help them twofold: firstly, in coping with the anxiety of suffering alopecia areata and secondly, exercise/relaxation tends to avoid the build-up of stress that's considered the 'trigger' to hair loss.

Q70 Why do I see more hair come out when I use a conditioner. Is it the conditioner that pulls the hair out?

The 'rake-like' action of your fingers when applying conditioner through your hair is similar to combing and brushing. In effect you're clearing your natural 'fall-out'. This has nothing to do with the conditioner itself.

Q71 Is it true that hair and nails are made of the same material?

Yes, they are both protein structures. Hair growth disorders often coexist with problem nails. Being essentially the same material they will both react negatively to systemic disease and nutritional deficiencies.

Q72 How often should I shampoo?

Daily is healthiest unless you have extremely dry hair when a maximum of three times a week is sufficient.

Q73 Should I brush my hair directly after shampooing (when it is wet), or is it best to wait until it has dried off?

Hair is at its most vulnerable when wet. I strongly advise a comb, particularly when de-tangling directly after shampooing. A brush is definitely best kept for when your hair has at least been towel dried.
   See page 49 (part B) for the safest combing/de-

tangling technique to employ and take a look at Question 74 for details on the healthiest types of combs and brushes to use.

Q74 What sort of combs and brushes are recommended?

The best combs have wide-set (but not sharp) teeth and should be made of vulcanised rubber. Never use metal or cheap plastic combs, these can damage hair.

A good brush is one with wide-spaced, smooth plastic bristles with ball-shaped tips; avoid using brushes with square or pointed tips and avoid metal or very sharp bristle brushes. Vent brushes are recommended if you blow-dry your hair on a regular basis. These have small spaces cut into them that allow the heat emitted from hairdryers to disperse evenly throughout the hair, therefore reducing both the blow-drying time and the chances of any subsequent hair damage.

These types of combs and brushes are readily found in trichological practices, high street chemists and some hairdressing salons (for best brushes for babies take a look at Question 34).

Q75 What foods are best for healthy hair growth?

Following a diet balanced in proteins, minerals, vitamins, fats, carbohydrates and water will ensure a healthy body system along with healthy hair growth. However, to specifically target hair growth the following foods should be included in your diet regularly.

Foods to include in your diet	What they contain to aid hair growth
Green vegetables	Iron Vitamin A Vitamin B1 (thiamine) Vitamin B2 (riboflavin) Vitamin B3 (niacin) Vitamin B5 (pantothenic acid) Vitamin B6 (pyridoxine) Folic acid Vitamin C
Dried fruits	Iron Vitamin A
Eggs	Vitamin B1 (thiamine) Vitamin B2 (riboflavin) Vitamin B5 (pantothenic acid) Vitamin B6 (pyridoxine) Biotin Folic acid Vitamin B12 (cobalamin) Essential fatty acids Protein Amino acids: tyrosine, cysteine and lyseine
Poultry	Protein Amino acid: lyseine Essential fatty acids
Fish	Protein Vitamin B1 (thiamine) Vitamin B3 (niacin) Vitamin B5 (pantothenic acid) Vitamin B6 (pyridoxine) Essential fatty acids

Citrus fruits	Vitamin C
Red meats	Iron
Protein
Amino acids: lyseine and tyrosine
Vitamin B1 (thiamine)
Vitamin B2 (riboflavin)
Vitamin B3 (niacin)
Vitamin B5 (pantothenic acid)
Biotin
Folic acid
Vitamin B12 (cobalamin)
Pulses	Iron
Protein
Amino acid: tyrosine
Whole grain produce	Vitamin B5 (pantothenic acid)
Folic acid
Zinc
Protein
Amino acid: lyseine
Vegetable oils	Vitamin E

As well as eating nutritious foods, another extremely important factor for healthy hair growth is not to skip meals. Eat three times a day, avoiding gaps of five hours or more between meals. Of course, for your hair as well as the rest of your system, make sure you drink plenty of water.

Menopausal women suffering hair thinning should make an extra effort to include or increase their intake of phytoestrogens in their diet. Phytoestrogens are thought to boost flagging oestrogen levels, which will assist healthier hair growth. Good sources are:

- lentils;
- rye bread;
- soya beans;
- chick peas;
- fruit;
- vegetables;
- red clover, a perennial herb that is available as a food supplement.

Q76 I have just turned forty. When will I start to go grey? And is there a treatment?

You can start to go 'grey' (or more specifically, white) any time from one to a hundred years of age, depending on your genetic make up. Melanocytes (pigment-producing cells) responsible for the colour of our hair are pre-set to halt production at a certain point in time. To get a clearer idea of when this might happen to you, take a look at other members of your family.

There's no proven treatment for this common 'problem' as of yet, although the amino acid tyrosine may aid pigment production. Therefore check the food sources of tyrosine under Question 75. Supplements containing this particular amino acid are available through trichological practices and health food shops (and don't forget, hair colourants can always save the day!).

6

Myths

As a trichologist I often get asked questions that revolve around common hair myths or old wives' tales. A myth is to be found in every one of the following questions; the answers, on the other hand, will dispel them once and for all!

Q77 I shampoo my hair every day. Do you think that I'm encouraging more of my hair to fall out?

Take a look at page 22 where the hair growth cycle is explained; it is a natural phenomenon that a specific amount of hair is shed and replaced all of the time. It's a complete myth that the simple act of shampooing can influence the rate of hair shedding.

I have met a number of hair loss sufferers over the years who believed this old wives' tale, and, out of sheer dread, would avoid shampooing for days, weeks or even months! The problem here is that when they finally summoned up the courage to wash their hair, the accumulated 'shedding' was quite a shock, sending these individuals into complete turmoil (see also Question 56). Sadly, unless expert advice is sought and adhered to, this cycle is repeated over and over again, leading to severe anxiety and depression on the part of the hair loss sufferer.

Take a look at Question 72. For most hair types it is healthiest to shampoo daily. This maintains a clean, healthy scalp while adding extra body, shine and manageability, especially to thinning hair.

Q78 I shampoo every day. Am I stripping the natural oils from my scalp?

The production of scalp oil (or sebum) is a continuous process that is predominately governed by the hormonal system, not by shampooing, however frequent.

Q79 Could shampooing your hair in 'hard' water make it fall out?

A film of calcium salts may build up on your hair if you live in a hard water area. Fortunately, this won't encourage hair loss but it may lead to rather dull-looking hair; consult a qualified trichologist who will recommend a shampoo and conditioner that will take any such circumstances into account.

An additional factor with 'hard' water is that you may need to apply a lot of shampoo to create a decent foam or lather. However, the production of a vast amount of foam will not increase the cleaning efficacy of any type of shampoo and is therefore a worthless exercise and a waste of shampoo.

Q80 Is it true that if you pull one grey hair out of your scalp, three will grow in its place?

Genetic forces control when we go grey or rather, white. Melanocytes (pigment-producing cells) halt production at a predetermined time. Pulling a white hair out will have no effect on this process whatsoever (see Question 76).

Q81 My hair is naturally very thick and coarse. Am I therefore less likely to suffer male pattern baldness?

Hair texture has no bearing on your chances of developing hair loss. Many men can have genetically thick-textured hair, but find over a period of time that they are also genetically programmed to suffer male pattern baldness.

Q82 My hair is thinning; if I shave it off will it grow back thicker?

Reducing the length of your hair will not encourage thicker hair growth. However, I can see how this myth evolved. When hair is shaved, the stubble that re-grows will *feel* thicker simply because it feels prickly. This is because the tapered end of the hair shaft has been cut off, leaving a blunt hair shaft behind.

Q83 I suffer from male pattern baldness and in my younger days I was in the army; do you think the hats I had to wear destroyed my hair?

There is no way that a hat could cause male pattern baldness. Take a look at pages 3–4 for the mechanics behind this condition.

Q84 Would my hair grow thicker and faster if I brushed it a hundred times before going to bed every night?

Brushing will certainly stimulate the scalp and hair to some degree, although not to the extent of encouraging thicker or faster hair growth. It is worth remembering that excessive brushing may cause hair breakage.

Q85 Could shampooing or rinsing your hair regularly with freezing cold water promote hair growth?

No it couldn't, thankfully! The only time cool water is useful is when rinsing out hair conditioners. But even in these circumstances, luke warm is cold enough.

Q86 My parents tell me that all the hair gel and styling mousse I use will make my hair come out. Is this true?

Hairstyling products only stick or cling onto your hair shafts; they do not in any way hinder healthy hair growth or encourage hair loss. However, always ensure that you comb these agents out of your hair on a daily basis and shampoo regularly. A build-up of these products could cause dry/brittle hair and may cause an itchy scalp.

Q87 Are split ends really repairable?

Split ends are a consequence of the natural degeneration of the hair shafts that occur root to tip. By the time long hair is achieved the tips of the hair shafts fray and form 'fork-like' ends. This degeneration of hair is known as 'hair weathering'. Usual suspects such as brushing, hair dryers and bleaching are all influential factors.

The only way to be rid of split ends is to cut them off, but to avoid split ends from forming in the first place always trim your hair every four to six weeks, even if you are trying to grow it long. For more information see Question 26.

Q88 Have bald men more male hormones than men with full heads of hair?

Some disappointing news here I'm afraid! What determines male pattern baldness is the sensitivity of the hair follicles to male hormones, not necessarily the quantity of hormone. This sensitivity is predetermined by genetics.

Q89 Is it true that if a cow licked the bald spot on the top of my head my hair will grow back again?

I'm afraid there's no truth in this whatsoever!

Q90 Rubbing stinging nettles onto a bald scalp . . . will it or won't it encourage hair re-growth?

No it won't! One of my clients told me that one of his friends actually tried this and ended up in casualty with a severe skin reaction ... and yes, to this day he remains bald!

Q91 I love Marmite on bread and toast but I have heard that if you massage it into your scalp it will aid hair re-growth.

Marmite is a rich source of B complex vitamins that happen to be good for hair, but imagine how ghastly it would look stuck to your scalp! Not to mention how it would smell! The best way to absorb these vitamins would be to keep eating your Marmite sandwiches.

Q92 How about the one about bats urine . . . ?

Let's not go anywhere near that subject!

Q93 My grandmother keeps telling me to rinse my thinning hair in beer. She says that it will create stronger hair growth, is this true?

In your grandmother's time, beer was thought of as a setting agent as well as a thickening agent. After a woman's hair had been rinsed in beer (and once the hair had dried off), the hair shafts would remain stuck together in a thick mass. This mass of hair was then moulded into the desired hairstyle and an illusion of having thicker, more lustrous hair was created! This reaction was clearly only a superficial one; no positive effects of boosting stronger hair growth were ever reported!

Q94 My mother has warned me that once I start plucking my eyebrows they will grow back even thicker than before. Is she correct?

No. Quite the contrary, plucking actually traumatises hair follicles which in time results in weaker hair growth.

Q95 If you catch head lice does this mean you have dirty hair?

No! Refer to Questions 35 through to 38 for further information on this problem and its remedy.

Q96 I suffer hereditary male hair loss. If I stood on my head would my hair grow back again?

This idea has never had any scientific reality! Check back to Chapter 1, in particular Questions 5 and 11 for details of the most effective and indeed more efficient ways of dealing with male hair loss!

Q97 My grandfather, who is eighty-five, still has a full head of hair. He puts this down to the fact that he has always massaged oil into his scalp. He is advising me to do the same to ward off hair loss. I would certainly have a go if I thought it would work, but would it?

Your grandfather is obviously genetically programmed to keep his hair, a very lucky man indeed! I am afraid it would not have had anything to do with the application of oil.

7
Useful Contacts

To locate a qualified trichologist in your area contact:

The Institute of Trichologists
Ground Floor Office
24 Langroyd Road
London
SW17 7PL
Telephone: 08706 070602
Website: www.trichologists.org.uk
E-mail: admin@trichologists.org.uk

The Institute of Trichologists was founded in 1902 and is the main qualifying body and professional association for trichologists in the UK. The Institute can be contacted for a list of qualified trichologists who are based all over the UK, Ireland and abroad.

The International Association of Trichologists
Suite 919
185 Elizabeth Street
Sydney
NSW 2000
Australia
Telephone: (0061) 02 9267 1384
Website: www.trichology.edu.au

This Association was established in 1974 and has trained trichologists listed internationally.

Vanessa Bailey MIT MRIPH can be contacted via The Institute of Trichologists or visit www.vanessabailey.co.uk.

Index

5-alpha reductase 4
  inhibition 6

acne
  causing hair loss 71
  in women 17
adrenal glands 12–13
Afro-Caribbean hair 47–56
  care tips 49–50
  chemical relaxing 47, 50, 51–2, 54–5
  treatments causing problems 47–9
air travel and hair loss 36
almond oil 51
alopecia
  androgenetic *see* androgenetic alopecia
  areata 20, 44, 71–2, *72*
    in beard area 71
  in children 43–4
  occipital 37–8
  traction 49
  traumatic cosmetic 52–3, *53*
  universalis 9
anaemia causing hair loss 21, 25–6
anesthetics causing hair loss 20
anagen phase of hair growth 6, 22
  effluvium 19
  Regain use and 8
androgenetic alopecia
  female 16–19
  male 3–4, 9
androgens
  causing PCOS 17–18
  in HRT 23
anti-ageing hormone 12–13
anti-androgens
  for hair loss 28
  for PCOS 17–18
antibiotics 21
anti-cancer drugs *see* chemotherapy
anti-clotting drugs 21
anti-depressants 21
anti-fungal agents for ringworm 43
aqueous cream 51, 56

back-combing 29–30
baldness
  female pattern *see* female hair loss
  male pattern *see* male hair loss
bat's urine and hair growth 84
beard, bald patches in 70–1
beer and hair growth 84–5
bereavement causing hair loss 20
bleached hair
  after chemotherapy 62
  green tinge to 59
  sun care 5
blonde hair, green tinge to 59
blood circulation in scalp 58

blood tests 12, 34
    for hormone imbalance 26–7, 35
braiding 48, 50, 52, 55
brushes 32
    buying 74
    for children 39
brushing hair
    after shampooing 73–4
    and stimulation 82

calcium
    in hard water 80
    in relaxers 54
carbaryl lice treatment 43
castration for male pattern baldness 8
catagen phase of hair growth 22
cell turnover
    chemotherapy and 62–3
    in psoriasis 66
    in seborrhoeic dermatitis 64
chelating agents in shampoos 59
chemical relaxing of curly hair 47, 50, 51–2, 54–5
    no-lye types 54
chemotherapy causing hair loss 19, 62–3
children's hair 37–46
chlorine damage to hair 59
Climen 24
clippers 55–6
coal tar 38
coarse hair 81
coconut oil 51
cold caps during chemotherapy 62–3
cold water shampooing 82
colouring hair 30–3
    after chemotherapy 62
    to hide scars 67–8
    see also dyeing
combs 32
    after shampooing 73–4
    buying 74

for de-tangling 49
following regrowth of hair 62
hot comb pressing 48
for nit removal 41–2
conditioning treatments 28, 32
    for Afro-Caribbean hair 50
    for children 43, 44–5, 46
    hair loss and 73
    massaging into scalp, problems 50
    rinsing out 82
    scalp problems and 65
    technique 69
copper ions in swimming pools 59
counselling for trichotillomania 61
cover-up sprays 29, 68
cow's spit and hair growth 83
cradle cap 38–9, 65
creams, for psoriasis 67
curlers 49–50
curly hair, chemical relaxing 47, 50, 51–2, 54–5
cuticle damage 29–30, *31*, 31–2, 50, 59
cutting
    hair 32, 45–6, 83
    transplanted hair 11
Cyclogest 24
cyproterone acetate 24, 28

dandruff 63–5
    anti-dandruff shampoos 71
    diet and 60
dehydroepiandrosterone 12–13
dermatitis
    infantile seborrhoeic 38–9
    seborrhoeic 60, *63*, 63–5
de-scaling agent 38
desogestrel 18
de-tangling 45, 49
DHEA *see* dehydroepiandrosterone
DHT *see* dihydrotestosterone

diagnosis of hair loss 7
Dianette 18, 28
diet
   causing hair loss 12, 20, 25, 34
   causing smelly hair 46
   dandruff and 60
   for greying hair 77
   for healthy hair growth 74–7
dihydrotestosterone 3–4
   Propecia use and 8
doll's head graft 3, 10
drying hair 45
   Afro-Caribbean hair 52
dyeing transplanted hair 11
   see also colouring hair

eczema *see* dermatitis
exercise and hair loss 57
extensions 48
eyebrows, plucking 85

familial tendencies to hirsutism 27
female hair loss 15–36
   age of occurrence 24–5, 33
   causes 17–19
   genetics 16, 24, 35
   hair serums 30
   hormone imbalance and 26–7
   HRT and 23–4
   iron-deficiency and 21, 25–6
   lifestyle 36
   non-pattern loss 19–21
   pattern of loss 16, *17*
   percentage affected 25
   pregnancy and 21–2
   questionnaire for 34–5
   treatments 27–9
finasteride *see* Propecia
flutamide 28
follicular stimulating hormone
   serum levels 26–7
folliculitis nuchae 55–6, *56*
foods
   causing dandruff 60, 65

causing psoriasis 66–7
for healthy hair growth 74–7, 84
frizziness 30
FSH *see* follicular stimulating hormone

gels 65, 82
genetics
   psoriasis 66
   in seborrhoeic dermatitis 63–4
genetics of hair loss
   female 16, 24, 35
   male 9
gestodene 18
greying hair 77, 81
grooming, male 9
guanidine hydroxide in relaxers 54

hair
   braiding 48, 50, 52, 55
   breakage 31, 51–2, 82
   care checklists 9, 32–3, 49–50, 68–9, 75–6
   colouring 30–3
   frizziness 30
   growth 6, 45–6, 81
      brushing and 82
      cycle 22–3
      in fetus 37
      myths 79–86
      summertime 58
   loss, female *see* female hair loss
      male *see* male hair loss
   pulling out 60–2
   split ends 83
   straightening 48
   sun care 5, 32–3
   tangling 44–5
   texture 81
   weathering 83
hair bands/ties 32, 45, 70

hair creams, for Afro-Caribbean hair 50
hair curlers 49–50
hair extensions 48, 52, 53–4
hair follicles 3–4
  atrophy 66
  growth in summer 58
  infection 55–6
hair greases, for Afro-Caribbean hair 50
hair loss
  in Afro-Caribbeans 48–9, 53–4
  from chemotherapy 19, 62–3
  in children 43–4
  conditioning treatments and 73
  exercise and 57
  in females *see* female hair loss
  in males *see* male hair loss
  shampooing and 58–9, 79–80
hair mascaras 67–8
hair replacement, non-surgical 7
hair serums 30
hair transplants, surgical 3, 7, 10, *11*, 29
  for scars 68
hairdryer settings 32, 52
hairline recession 3
  in Afro-Caribbeans 52–3
  in children 46
  possible causes 11–12
hairpieces 29
  for scar areas 68
hard water and shampooing 80
hats and baldness 81–2
head lice 39–43, 85
hereditary hair thinning, male *see* inheritance of male hair loss
highlighted hair, sun care 5
hirsutism in women 17, 26–7
hormone replacement therapy 18, 23–4
hormones
  affecting hair follicles 3–4
  bald men and 83
  imbalance causing female hair loss 26–7, 35
  male steroid type 12–13
  puberty 46
hot comb pressing 48, 52–3
HRT *see* hormone replacement therapy
hyperthyroidism causing hair loss 21
hypnosis for trichotillomania 61
hypothyroidism causing hair loss 21

illness causing hair loss 12, 20
infantile seborrhoeic dermatitis 38–9
infection, with cradle cap 39
inheritance of male hair loss 4–5, 9
injury causing hair loss 20
Institute of Trichologists 87
International Association of Trichologists 87–8
iron supplementation 25–6
iron-deficiency causing hair loss 21, 25–6

lanolin 51
lanugo hair 37–8
LH *see* luteinizing hormone
libido improvement 13
lice 39–43, 85
lithium hydroxide in relaxers 54
long hair
  hair loss 70
  shampooing 69
  tangling 44–5
  thinning 70
luteinizing hormone serum levels 26–7

male hair loss 3–14
  age of occurrence 3, 5
  hair care and 9
  hair texture and 81

hats and 81–2
hormones and *see* hormones
how it happens 3–4
inheritance 4–5, 9
other causes 11–12
pattern of loss *4*
steroid hormones and 12–13
sun care 5
surgical hair transplants for *see* hair transplants, surgical
treatments 6–8
   coming off 8
   myths 85
   see also hair replacement, non-surgical; hair transplants, surgical
Marmite and hair growth 84
Marvelon 18
mascaras, hair 67–8
massaging scalp 69
   hair growth and 57–8, 86
   problems with conditioners 50
medication causing hair loss
   in females 16–17, 19, 21
   in males 12
medroxyprogesterone 24
melanocytes 77, 81
menopause
   diet 76–7
   and hair loss 16, 23–4
   scalp massage and 58
menstrual problems 17, 36
   anaemia from 25
metabolism and hair loss 21
micro-grafting 3, 10, *11*
minoxidil *see* Regaine
moisturisers, for Afro-Caribbean hair 50, 51, 56
mousses 65, 82

nail problems 73
nits 41–2
no-lye relaxers 54
norethisterone 18, 23
norgestrel 18, 23

occipital alopecia 37–8
oestrogen and hair loss 22, 23, 36
oil for scalp massage 86
olive oil for cradle cap 38
oral contraceptives and hair loss 18–19, 35
oral treatments 6

patch tests for colourants 33
PCOS *see* polycystic ovarian syndrome
permethrin lice treatment 42
phenothrin lice treatment 42
phytoestrogens in diet 76–7
pituitary gland hormones 27
pityrosporum ovale 64, 65
plucking eyebrows 85
polycystic ovarian syndrome 17–18
potassium in relaxers 54
pregnancy and hair loss 21–2
progesterone serum levels 26–7
progestogen
   in HRT 23
   natural 24
   -only oral contraceptives 18
Propecia 6
   coming off 8
   using with Regaine 8
psoriasis on scalp 66
puberty and hair loss 46
pulling out hair 60–2

questionnaire for female hair loss 34–5

razors 55–6
receding hairline *see* hairline recession
reducing agents in shampoos 59
Regaine 6, 27–8
   coming off 8
   using with Propecia 8
relaxers *see* chemical relaxing of curly hair

relaxation techniques for stress 72
retinoids 21
ringworm 43–4
Rogaine *see* Regaine
root lifting by back-combing 29–30

salicylic acid in shampoo 38
scalp
  condition in psoriasis 65–7
  condition in seborrhoeic dermatitis 63–5
  infection 55–6
  massaging 50, 57–8, 69, 86
  moisturising 50, 51
  scars 67–8
  sensitivity 50, 51
scalp mesh/net 7
scalp oil *see* sebum
scalp solutions for psoriasis 67
scars on scalp 67–8
sebaceous glands, at puberty 46
seborrhoeic dermatitis *see* dermatitis
sebum 46
  production 64, 80
sensitivity test for colourants 33
serums 30
shampoo
  for Afro-Caribbean hair 50
  anti-dandruff 71
  chelating agents in 59
  children's hair 38, 46
  daily 46
  for psoriasis 67
  reducing agents in 59
shampooing
  after swimming 59–60
  in cold water 82
  daily 80
  frequency 73
  hair loss and 58–9, 79–80
  in hard water 80

long hair 69, 70
scalp problems and 65
to stop build-up of products 82
techniques 68–9
shaved hair 81
shock causing hair loss 20
skin
  health improvement 13
  testing for colourants 33
  thinning following steroids 67
smelly hair 46
sodium hydroxide 47, 54
sodium thiosulfate 59
spironolactone 28
split ends 83
steaming hair 49
steroid creams for scalps 67
stinging nettles and hair growth 84
straightening hair 48
stress
  causing hair loss 12, 20
  causing alopecia areata 72
  causing trichotillomania 60
  causing psoriasis 66–7
styling
  Afro-Caribbean hair 52
  transplanted hair 11
summertime and hair growth 58
sun care
  bald patches 5
  hair 5, 32–3
sunburn prevention 5
surgery causing hair loss 20
swimming and hair damage 59

tangling 44–5
telogen phase of hair growth 6, 22–3, 37–8, 58–9
  effluvium, acute 19–20, 36
    chronic 20
  during pregnancy 22
testosterone
  DHEA conversion to 12–13

and hair growth 4, 13
  serum levels 26–7
testosterone and hair growth 4
tetrasodium EDTA 59
thyroid gland problems causing
  hair loss 21
thyroxine 21
tinted hair, sun care 5
topical treatments 6, 28
traction hair loss 48
treatments for hair loss 6–8, 27–9
  see also hair replacement, non-surgical; hair transplants, surgical
trichologists 7
  for female hair loss 28–9

trichotillomania 60–2
trimming *see* cutting
trisodium thiosulfate 59
tyrosine 77

ultraviolet therapy in psoriasis 67

vellus hairs 4

water intake 76
weight gain in women 17
well-being improvement 13
wigs 29
Wood's Lamp 43

Yasmin 18

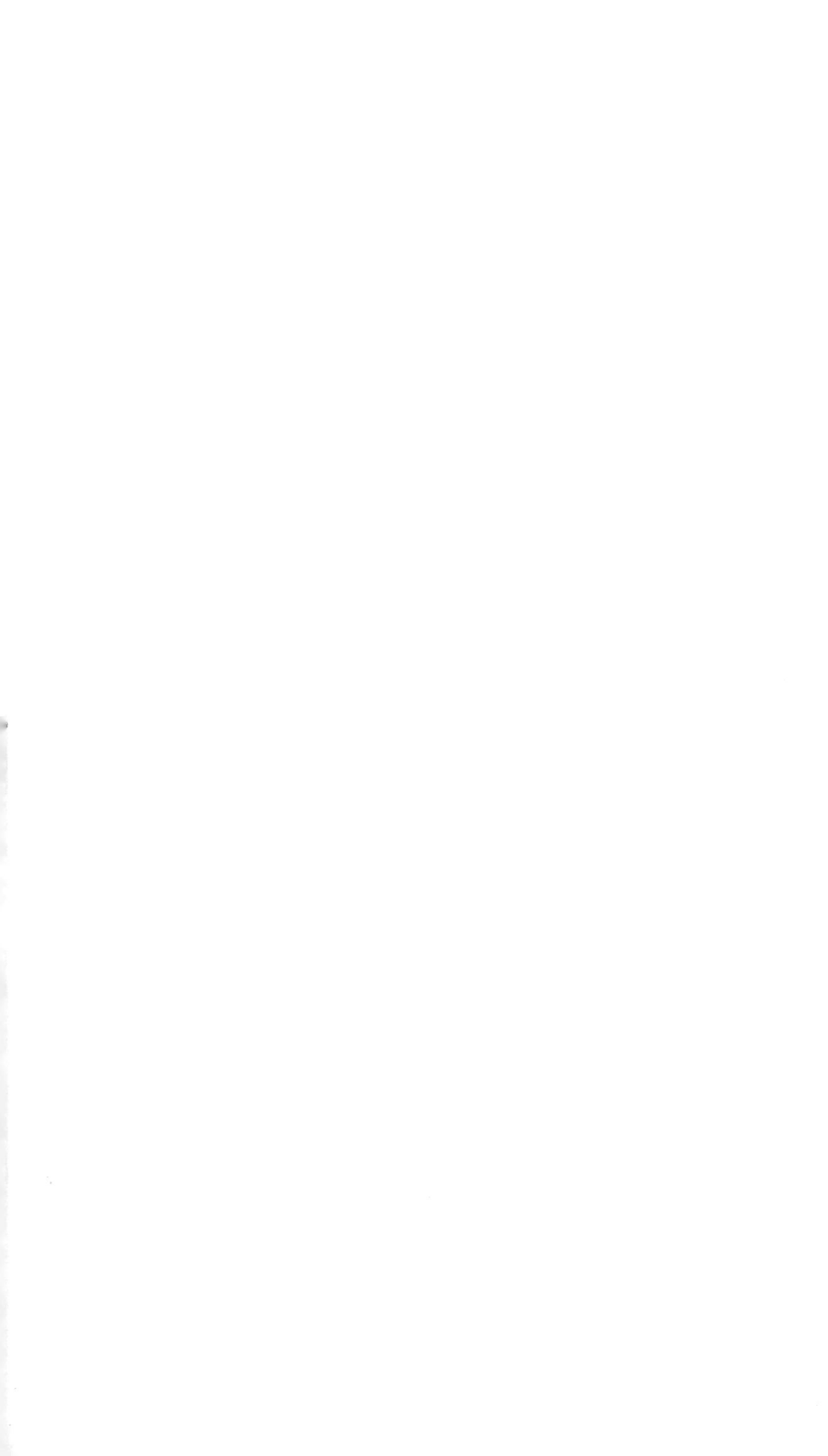

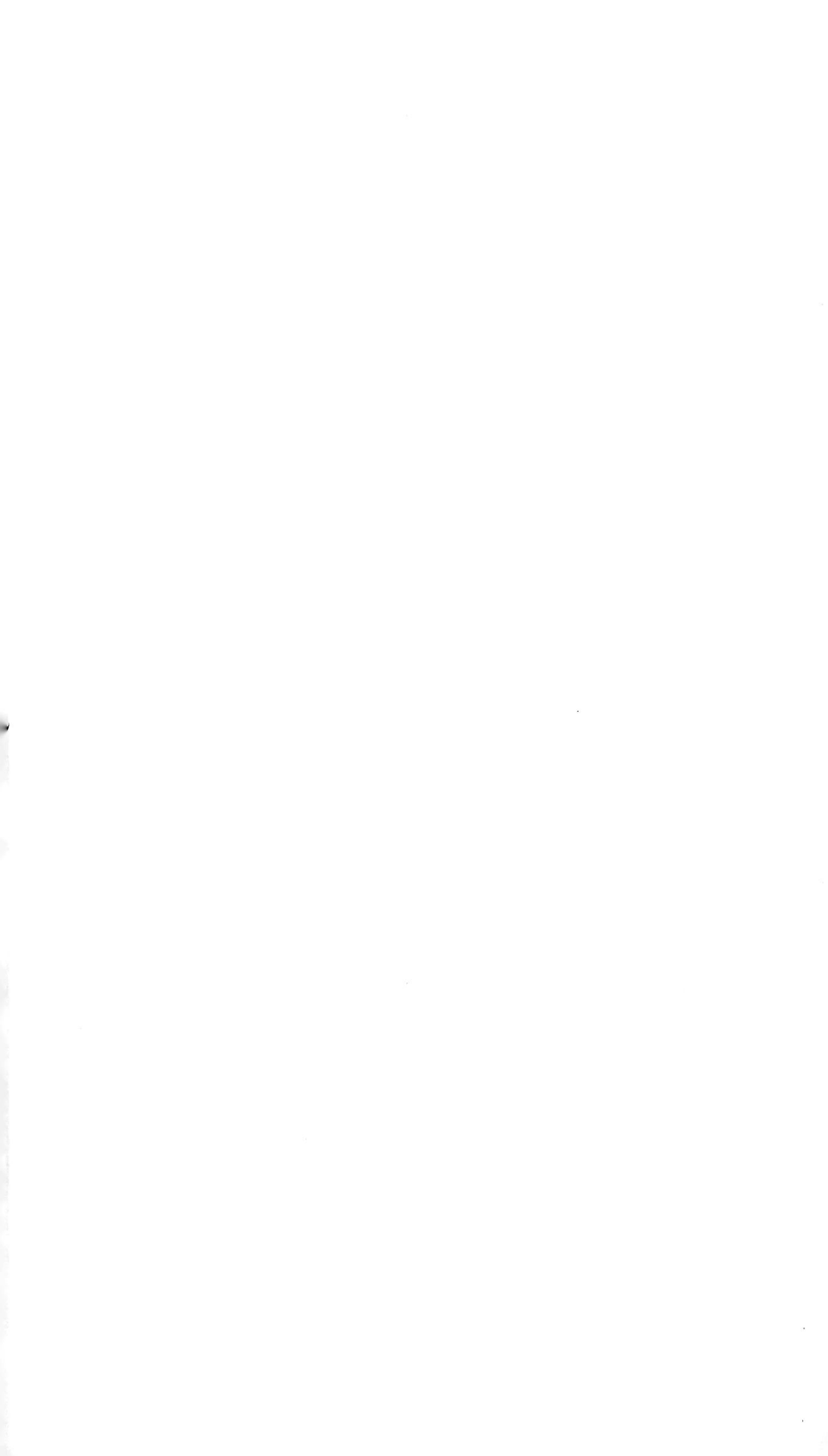